Celiac Disease

Also by Sylvia Llewelyn Bower, RN

What Nurses Know . . . Gluten-Free Lifestyle

Celiac Disease

A Guide to Living with Gluten Intolerance

Second Edition

Sylvia Llewelyn Bower, RN

with

Mary Kay Sharrett, MS, RD, LD, CNSD,
and Steve Plogsted, PHARMD

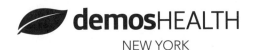

NEW YORK

Visit our website at www.demoshealth.com

ISBN: 978-1-936303-63-2

e-book ISBN: 978-1-617052-06-4

Acquisitions Editor: Julia Pastore

Compositor: diacriTech

Medical information provided by Demos Health, in the absence of a visit with a health care professional, must be considered as an educational service only. This book is not designed to replace a physician's independent judgment about the appropriateness or risks of a procedure or therapy for a given patient. Our purpose is to provide you with information that will help you make your own health care decisions.

The information and opinions provided here are believed to be accurate and sound, based on the best judgment available to the authors, editors, and publisher, but readers who fail to consult appropriate health authorities assume the risk of injuries. The publisher is not responsible for errors or omissions. The editors and publisher welcome any reader to report to the publisher any discrepancies or inaccuracies noticed.

Library of Congress Cataloging-in-Publication Data

Bower, Sylvia Llewelyn.

  Celiac disease : a guide to living with gluten intolerance / Sylvia Llewelyn Bower, RN with Mary Kay Sharrett, MS, RD, LD, CNSD, and Steve Plogsted, PharmD[M01]. —Second edition.

     pages cm

  Includes bibliographical references and index.

  ISBN 978-1-936303-63-2

  1. Celiac disease—Popular works. 2. Gluten-free diet—Popular works. I. Sharrett, Mary Kay. II. Plogsted, Steve. III. Title.

  RC862.C44B69 2014

  616.3'99--dc23

                              2014014102

Special discounts on bulk quantities of Demos Health books are available to corporations, professional associations, pharmaceutical companies, health care organizations, and other qualifying groups. For details, please contact:

Special Sales Department
Demos Medical Publishing, LLC
11 West 42nd Street, 15th Floor
New York, NY 10036
Phone: 800-532-8663 or 212-683-0072
Fax: 212-941-7842
E-mail: specialsales@demosmedical.com

Printed in the United States of America by McNaughton & Gunn.

14 15 16 17 18 / 5 4 3 2 1

This book is dedicated to my husband Jack Bower who has been by my side and encouraged me through it all.

Contents

Foreword

Celiac disease is now considered to be one of the most common chronic conditions affecting mankind and occurs in about 1% of the general population in the United States. While it has been gratifying to see the diagnosis made more frequently in the past two decades, there are still many people with celiac disease who remain undiagnosed or go for prolonged periods with symptoms before the condition is recognized. Confirming a diagnosis of celiac disease can bring relief to those who have suffered unexplained symptoms for long periods of time but may lead to a host of new concerns that go with the major lifestyle changes that occur with treatment. Maintaining a strict gluten-free diet for life is essential for the health and well-being of people with celiac disease. A gluten-free diet can be cumbersome to follow, increase the cost of living, and impose new restrictions on one's lifestyle. For these reasons it is important to be certain of the diagnosis and not confuse celiac disease with other "gluten" sensitive conditions for which such strict adherence to the diet may not be necessary.

The second edition of *Celiac Disease: a Guide to Living with Gluten Intolerance* by Sylvia Llewelyn Bower is both timely and a delight to read. The author takes one through a brief history of celiac disease before describing the variable clinical manifestations that make the condition so unique and interesting. Tests to identify those who might have celiac disease are covered and the importance of confirming the diagnosis by means of an intestinal biopsy is emphasized.

There is a chapter on the gluten-free diet written by Mary Kay Sharrett, who is one of the foremost experts on the subject in the United States. An additional chapter on gluten in medications, written by another renowned authority on the subject, Steve Plogsted, covers an important and often forgotten potential source of inadvertent gluten ingestion.

The book is full of valuable information covering topics that are seldom addressed but are so important to those who live the life of celiac disease. "Tackling the Emotional Side of Celiac Disease" and "Raising a Child with Celiac Disease" are particularly helpful. Numerous personal anecdotal stories are included that highlight some of the issues people with celiac disease deal with both before and after the diagnosis is made. These stories not only illustrate some of the difficulties and frustrations experienced, but offer hope to others when they read how the adversities were overcome.

The book concludes with helpful tips on dining out and provides a brief insight into some potential future alternative forms of treatment. Best of all is the long list of gluten-free recipes that will delight many who struggle to live with the diet. This is a must read for both those who are newly diagnosed and the "old hands" who will find a lot of additional useful information that can make life with celiac disease seem all the more enjoyable.

Ivor Hill, MD
Medical Director
Celiac Disease Center
Nationwide Children's Hospital
Columbus, Ohio

Preface

This book is written in the sincere attempt to offer new and vital information to individuals diagnosed with celiac disease (CD) or non-celiac gluten sensitivity (NCGS). Knowledge will set us free. Family members and health care professionals also will gain insight and information to guide and encourage newly diagnosed individuals.

Each chapter is written to inform, challenge, and encourage the individual with CD or NCGS. We know now that this population is large. Recent studies have revealed how common CD is. It is estimated that there could be 3,000,000 people with the disease in the United States alone. The incidence of CD in families is 1 in 22 for first-degree relatives (parents and siblings) and 1 in 39 in second-degree relatives (grandparents, aunts, uncles, and cousins).

Writing this new edition, I have come to appreciate how much new research has been done. When this book was first written there were about two to three new research papers each month. Now there are as many as several hundred monthly. The medical profession has taken giant steps forward in its ability to diagnose and treat CD. This condition was considered "rare" as recently as the year 2000. Many would have to endure symptoms for 15 to 20 years before receiving a diagnosis. This was devastating. Currently, there are also several clinical trials for various treatments of CD. These are important as these trials are our best opportunity to improve outcomes and treatment methods.

Despite these advances, many unanswered questions remain:

* What triggers the body to suddenly reject the proteins in wheat, barley, and rye?
* Are there ways to prevent CD or NCGS?
* What is the relationship between CD and NCGS and other autoimmune disorders? Other health conditions?
* What are the systemic consequences of CD and NCGS?
* What are the economic consequences of CD and NCGS?

The good news is that we are getting closer to answering these questions each day as researchers and physicians around the world dedicate themselves to understanding this disease. To name just a few:

> Dr. Ivor Hill at Nationwide Children's Hospital, Columbus, Ohio
> Dr. Alessio Fasano at Massachusetts General Hospital, Boston
> Dr. Joseph Murray at the Mayo Clinic, Rochester, Minnesota
> Dr. Peter Green at Columbia University, New York
> Dr. Stefano Guandalini at the University of Chicago, Illinois
> Dr. Alberto Rubio-Tapia at the Mayo Clinic, Rochester, Minnesota

In addition, the American Celiac Disease Alliance continues to advocate for our rights, successfully working with Congress and the FDA to enact food labeling legislation, and the National Institutes of Health supports important CD research, resulting in much of the current information and data on CD included in this book.

I hope this book provides you with solace and comfort and empowers you to improve your health.

Acknowledgments

A personal thanks goes to the Gluten-Free Gang of Central Ohio. This dynamic support group is filled with positive, supportive people who were very willing to share their stories so that others would benefit from them. To name names would be endless.

To my sister, Elizabeth Elmquist, an editor with experience, I am eternally grateful for your many hours of work and perseverance in "massaging" my words to help them come out right.

To Demos Health for being willing to publish this text so that it could benefit those who have been diagnosed with celiac disease (CD) or have a family member or child that could benefit from this information.

To the researchers who spend many hours in doing prevalence studies, clinical studies, and clinical practice and continue to determine ways that will allow for more comprehensive diagnosis and treatment of CD. You have our future in your hands.

CHAPTER 1

What Is Celiac Disease?

Courage is the first of human qualities because it is the quality which guarantees all the others.
—Winston Churchill

Celiac disease (CD) has gone from the depths of the darkest pits of ignorance into the light of knowledge within the last fifteen years. "For wisdom will enter your heart and knowledge will be pleasant to your soul," according to Proverbs 2:10. Knowing all about CD will empower you to discuss it, share your information and experiences, teach about it, and, above all, live with it!

CD is an autoimmune disorder that stimulates T cells—white blood cells essential for healthy immunity—to inflame the mucosa or lining of the small bowel and destroy the villi in the small intestine, preventing the absorption of nutrients from food into the bloodstream. We are not born with CD, but it occurs in people who are genetically predisposed and can be triggered by a viral or bacterial infection, pregnancy, or the consumption of the protein gluten present in the grains of wheat, barley, and rye. There are about 3,000,000 people with CD in the United States, and it is found in 1% of the population worldwide

No expensive pills, elixirs, lotions, or injections can heal the body of a person with CD. Understanding CD and following a strict diet that excludes wheat, barley, and rye and all their derivatives are the only ways that people with CD can eliminate their symptoms. After being diagnosed, it is possible to regain your health. Each person is responsible for following the diet and ultimately eliminating the symptoms. However, it is dangerous to go on a gluten-free diet (GFD) before you have been diagnosed, because then a diagnosis cannot be made.

Our goal is to help you understand CD and gluten intolerance. We hope that this book will provide the information and knowledge that you need to make good decisions about your health and have the courage to help others understand what CD really entails.

History of CD

Though awareness of CD has become more widespread in recent years, there is evidence that the disease affected people as early as the first century AD. One of the earliest cases of CD was reported in the August 2010 issue of the *Journal of Clinical Gastroenterology*:

> A case of a young woman [who] died in Italy during the first century AD is presented. She had short height (140 cm), clinical history of anemia, and a decreased bone mass with evidence of osteoporosis and bone fragility. The archeological artifacts from the tomb, and with the quality of burial architecture, suggests the tomb was built for a rich person in an area with extensive culture of wheat. The wellness of the area is supported by the lack of other bodies found with signs of malnutrition. Clinical presentation and the possible continuous exposure to wheat seem to suggest a case of celiac disease. This case could be the first case of this condition since the one described by Aretaeus of Cappadocia in 250 BC and could be helpful to clarify the phylogenetic tree [the beginning] of celiac disease.

The agricultural revolution of the Neolithic period generated a whole new battery of food antigens previously unknown to man, according to Dr. Stefano Guandalini of the Celiac Research Center at the University of Chicago. Besides all of the new grains like wheat and barley, this included protein from the milk of cows, goats, and donkeys, as well as bird's eggs. This was the beginning of wheat and dairy allergies, food intolerances, and CD. Unrecognized and untreated, these allergies and CD resulted in many deaths from malnutrition and possibly cancer as we now know celiacs have an increased risk of developing that disease.

The term "celiac" is derived from the Greek word *koiliakos* meaning "suffering of the bowel" and was introduced in about 250 AD by Aretaeus of Cappadocia. He recognized that there were children who were malnourished even though they were being fed a nourishing diet. He seemed to know that it was food related. However, he could not determine what caused the disorder or how to treat it.

It was not until the 19th century that Dr. Mathew Baillie published his observations on CD as a "chronic diarrheal disorder causing malnutrition and characterized by a gas distended abdomen." He also stated that his patients benefited from eating rice.

In 1888, Dr. Samuel Gee, of the Great Ormond Street Hospital for Children in the United Kingdom, presented clinical studies of CD including both children and adults. Dr. Gee prophetically said in his presentation, "To regulate the food is the main part of treatment. The allowance of farinaceous food [food containing starch] must be small, but if the patient can be cured at all, it must be by means of diet." Dr. Gee also documented improvement in a patient when introduced to a GFD who suffered relapse when gluten was reintroduced.

Dr. Gee was one of many physicians of his time to experiment with diets to relieve the symptoms of CD. Sir Fredrick Sill and Dr. John Howland proposed a three-stage diet where carbohydrates were introduced in the last stage of the diet. A "banana diet" theory, known as the diet for people with CD, was introduced in 1924 by Dr. Sydney V. Hass. The banana diet restricted carbohydrates (with the exception of ripe bananas) and fat. Typical foods for a child with CD on the diet included: albumin milk, pot cheese, bananas (as many as the child would take, usually four to eight each day), oranges, vegetables, gelatin, and meat. He observed ten children in his practice suffering from CD. Eight of the ten children went on a banana diet and two did not go on the diet. The children on the banana diet lived while the two children not on the banana diet died. This treatment was accepted for several decades.

One of the biggest advances in CD research happened in 1953 when Dr. Willem Karel Dicke wrote his doctoral thesis for the University of Utrecht. He predicted that the ingestion of wheat proteins was specifically the cause of CD and not carbohydrates. During World War II there was a tremendous bread shortage, especially in Europe because this is where the majority of the land fighting occurred. The health of the children with CD improved dramatically in the countries that experienced the shortage. When the allied planes started dropping bread, the same children's health quickly deteriorated. No one dared to doubt Dr. Dicke's doctoral thesis with this kind of evidence to back up his theory. These early studies followed CD in children, but it was also prevalent in adults.

In the 1950s and 1960s, increased interest in CD led researchers to discover relationships between CD, dermatitis herpetiformis (a skin disease of intensely itchy lesions), and numerous neurological disorders including epilepsy, cerebral calcifications, and peripheral neuropathy. Over the next 20 years, researchers improved the procedures for diagnosing the disease. In the 1980s, Dr. Guandalini and a panel of experts from the European society of Pediatric Gastroenterology, Hepatology, and Nutrition found that a single biopsy from the small intestine could detect the disease with 95% accuracy. This is the way CD was diagnosed for the next 20 years. In 1998 Gastroenterologist and researcher Detlef Schuppnan discovered that gluten in the intestines of people with celiac disease provokes the release of the enzyme transglutaminase and antibodies that regulate it. In 2000, Dr. Alessio Fasano's team at the Center for Celiac Disease developed an enzyme-linked immunosorbent assay (ELISA) that is used today as the initial diagnostic tool for blood screening that is 98% specific for celiac disease.

The history of CD is still being written today as new research continues. There is much we still don't know about this disease. The evolution of grains, the environment, and genetic factors all play a role. It's important to remember that CD is *not* a new disease, even though recent increases in familiarity may make it seem so. The more informed that you are about the history of CD, the easier it will be for you to educate your family, friends, and community, and raise awareness about the need for continued research.

What Is Celiac Disease?

CD is defined as a multisystem disorder that causes the body's immune system to respond to the protein in certain grains. The immune system builds antibodies against these proteins and attacks the intestinal lining or mucosa, causing inflammation and damage to the villi—hair-like structures on the lining of the small intestine. The wheat-type grains have protein complexes called *gliadin* that are harmful to people with CD. The barley-type grains have protein complexes called *hordein*, and rye has protein complexes called *secalin*. The chemical make-up of the gliadin, hordein, and secalin cause the body to have an immune reaction. It is still not understood why these grains do this. Gluten is found in other grains, such as corn, yet it causes no ill effects to CD patients.

The harmful forms of gluten are found in these grains and grain-derived products:

* Barley
* Couscous

* Durham
* Einkorn
* Emmer
* Farro
* Graham
* Kamut
* Malt
* Matzo
* Oats (unless gluten free)
* Orzo
* Rye
* Seitan
* Semolina
* Spelt
* Sprouted barley
* Sprouted wheat
* Teriyaki sauce (unless wheat-free)
* Triticale
* Udon
* Wheat

Avoid all regular baking flours, breads, pasta, pastries, and desserts made with the above grains and products.

In the digestive process, chewed food, mixed with saliva, goes from the mouth, into the esophagus, and enters the stomach, where gastric juices mix with the food. The food continues to travel into the small intestine. Nutrition from the food is absorbed through small projections, called villi, on the surface of the small intestine. The villi absorb the nutrition from the digesting food.

In CD, the gluten (protein) in certain grains causes the body to produce *endomysial antibodies* (EMA). An antibody, also known as an immunoglobulin (Ig), is a large Y-shape protein used by the immune system to identify and neutralize foreign objects. There are two varieties of EMA antibodies, EMA IgA and EMA IgG. These antibodies create an inflammatory process that destroys the villi (Figure 1-1). Previously, this

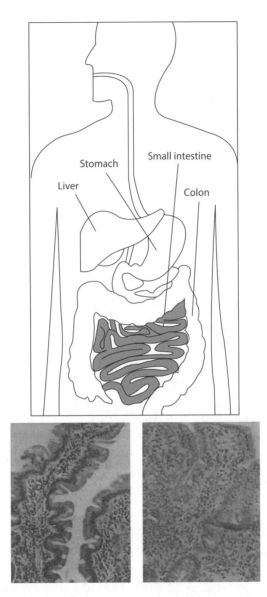

Figure 1-1. (Top) The digestive system. (Reprinted from "Celiac Disease" at the National Digestive Diseases Information Clearing House, http://digestive.niddk.nih.gov/DDISEASES/pubs/celiac) (Bottom) On the left is a normal villus that has indentations to absorb nutrients. On the right, the fingerlike projections are gone and the surface is basically flat and would have difficulty absorbing nutrients.

destruction was thought to be gluten-sensitive enteropathy or CD, gluten intolerance, gluten sensitivity, or even possibly a wheat allergy. The most recent information from the University of Chicago indicates that *only* CD causes villi destruction. *The other conditions do not.*

When the villi are destroyed, absorption is disturbed and nutrients from food will not enter the body. Food will continue to pass through the large intestine and be eliminated. The entire body may show symptoms because it is not receiving enough fuel to function.

The age of onset varies from infancy to the elderly, and the symptoms can be very subtle or obvious. An infant may show symptoms when he or she is introduced to grains at an early age. The symptoms may include diarrhea, constipation, foul-smelling stools, fatigue, slow growth pattern, irritability, and even a swollen belly from malnutrition. An older adult frequently presents with anemia from no apparent cause. It is not known why one person may develop CD at six months and another doesn't show symptoms until they are in their golden years. The average age of diagnosis, based on statistics, is between 40 and 60. However, one commonality exists for each individual diagnosed with this disease: No one is sure what triggers the disease. Some statistics show pregnancy, a virus, or stress may be the trigger, but no clear cause is obvious.

CD was, until the last few years, thought to be very rare in the United States. Few physicians realized its potential impact or researched its prevalence. Dr. Alessio Fasano, who came from Italy to the University of Maryland in 1993, reasoned that if 1 in 150 in Italy are prone to CD, then the United States, with its large European heritage, should have a high prevalence. Through research conducted at the Center for Celiac Research, which he founded in 1996, he discovered a prevalence rate of 1 in 133 persons. This would suggest that approximately three million U.S. residents have CD. The research indicates that the worldwide prevalence is 1 in 250.

Symptoms

The symptoms of CD may be varied and hard to define. The individual with CD may know he or she "feels bad" and realize that something is wrong, but be unaware of what to do about it. Some with CD may not know they have the disease and exhibit no symptoms and as many as 60% of people with CD may exhibit non-classic symptoms. The classic signs are fatigue, listlessness, diarrhea, and weight loss. If any of these persist for more than a few months, your doctor will usually order a blood test. The most common result of such testing is iron-deficiency anemia. This anemia is caused by the body not absorbing iron from the food that is eaten. In CD, the damage to the intestine may be so great that iron cannot be absorbed, and it is then possible that other nutrients, such as calcium and protein, also are not being properly absorbed.

> Celiac disease is a very common disorder, and most people with the disease have the silent form. These individuals are usually identified through screening of at-risk groups.
> —Dr. Peter Green

Because of the variety of symptoms presented, the disease is often overlooked by physicians in this age of the medical specialist. A patient may consult a psychiatrist, psychologist, or mental health social worker for symptoms of irritability, depression, and behavior changes. An orthopedic specialist or rheumatologist may be consulted for joint pain, bone pain, or osteoporosis. A dentist will see the individual for symptoms of dental enamel hypoplasia and sores in the mouth, but be unaware of his patient's other physical symptoms. An allergist may discover lactose intolerance or an allergy to milk or wheat. A dermatologist may be asked to treat the painful itching skin rash but, unless the skin is biopsied for dermatitis herpetiformis, CD will go undiagnosed because doctors do not usually associate diet with skin rashes. A hematologist may find that the person suffers from anemia of unknown origin. A neurologist will treat seizures or unsteady walking (ataxia), but may not be able to discover a clear reason for the episode because the patient's electroencephalogram does not show brain lesions.

> One form of CD causes very itchy, scaly skin lesions. When the skin is biopsied, CD can be identified through the antibodies present. This is called *dermatitis herpetiformis*, and it also causes the intestinal damage described in Figure 1-1. (See Chapter 3)

The family practitioner will have on file the symptoms of abdominal pain, bloating, constipation, diarrhea, chronic fatigue, gas, or perhaps type 1 diabetes. However, if the physician is not familiar with CD, the referral to a gastro-enterologist, which should be the first step toward a correct diagnosis, might not be made.

It is easy to see how the medical community might diagnose this individual as a hypochondriac. Many with CD have traveled from doctor to doctor, seeking relief from single symptoms when, if the pieces of the CD puzzle were only put together, their problem could be diagnosed easily.

> According to Ann Whelan of *Gluten-Free Living* and The National Institutes of Health (NIH), the following individuals should be tested for CD:
>
> * Those with classic symptoms of chronic diarrhea, malabsorption, weight loss, abdominal distention
> * Those with short stature, delayed puberty, iron-deficiency anemia, recurrent fetal loss, infertility

(continued)

> *(continued)*
>
> ✳ Those with irritable bowel syndrome, persistent aph-
> thous stomatitis (cold sores), autoimmune diseases,
> peripheral neuropathy, cerebellar ataxia, dental enamel
> hypoplasia
>
> Populations at risk include individuals with type I diabetes
> mellitus, first- and second-degree relatives of individuals
> with CD, individuals with Turner syndrome, and those
> with Down or Williams syndromes.

Self-Assessment

Use this assessment to help identify your symptoms and
determine if you should see your doctor for a diagnosis of
CD. If you have three of these symptoms in one category or
ten on the whole assessment, you should ask your doctor
for a celiac profile test. At that point, *do not* stop eating
gluten. Your doctor will need to see how the gluten in your
daily diet affects your body.

**SELF-ASSESSMENT TO EVALUATE FOR CELIAC
DISEASE**

	Always present	Occasionally	Never
GENERALIZED SYMPTOMS			
Fatigue			
Headache			
Joint pain			
Hair loss			
Heart palpitations			

(continued)

SELF-ASSESSMENT TO EVALUATE FOR CELIAC DISEASE *(continued)*

	Always present	Occasionally	Never
Shortness of breath			
Iron deficiency anemia			
Weight loss			

GASTROINTESTINAL

	Always present	Occasionally	Never
Diarrhea			
Constipation			
Bloating			
Reflux (heartburn)			
Abdominal pain			
Increased gas after eating			
Bulky or lose stools			
Irritable bowel			

SKIN

	Always present	Occasionally	Never
Itchy rash on elbows, knees			
Blistering rash			

NERVOUS SYSTEM

	Always present	Occasionally	Never
Numbness and tingling of feet and hands			
Difficulty with balance			
Depression			
Anxiety			
Behavioral changes			

(continued)

SELF-ASSESSMENT TO EVALUATE FOR CELIAC DISEASE (*continued*)

	Always present	Occasionally	Never
REPRODUCTIVE SYSTEM			
Infertility			
Still birth			
Recurrent abortion			
Preterm birth			
Low birth weight			
Cesarean section			
Endometriosis			
Pelvic pain			
Severe menstrual cramps			
Missed menstrual periods			
MOUTH			
Dental enamel problems			
Aphthous ulcers (canker sores)			
STRUCTURAL			
Osteopenia			
Osteoporosis (fractured or thin bones)			
Other bone deficiencies			
Fibromyalgia			

(*continued*)

SELF-ASSESSMENT TO EVALUATE FOR CELIAC DISEASE (*continued*)

	Always present	Occasionally	Never
Low calcium			
Joint pain			

CHILDREN TWO AND ABOVE

	Always present	Occasionally	Never
Diarrhea			
Constipation			
Short stature			
Delayed puberty			
Diabetes type I			
Down syndrome			
Delayed growth			

INFANTS

	Always present	Occasionally	Never
Chronic diarrhea			
Swollen belly			
Weight loss			
Pain			
Failure to thrive			
Down syndrome			

OTHER AUTOIMMUNE DISEASES

	Always present	Occasionally	Never
Fibromyalgia			
Hypothyroidism			
Sjögren's syndrome			
Multiple sclerosis			
Lupus erythematosus			
Insulin-dependent diabetes (type I)			

Celiac Disease vs. Non-Celiac Gluten Sensitivity

The large increase, interest, and use of the GFD has had a profound effect on the gluten-free world. The GFD has become popular and for many has become a way of life, whether they have a diagnosis of CD or not. According to Dr. Alessio Fasano, gluten is a toxic grain that most individuals have difficulty digesting. The fragments left in the intestinal tract can lead to inflammation for many people. However, there is a definite difference between CD and non-celiac gluten sensitivity (NCGS).

CD is an immune-mediated inflammation of the small intestine caused by the proteins in wheat, barley, and rye in genetically sensitive individuals. NCGS is characterized by gastrointestinal symptoms or other symptoms that respond positively to a GFD. The primary difference between these two conditions is that those with NCGS show no biological changes to the small intestine. When those with NCGS are biopsied, they show no evidence of inflammation or destruction of the villi.

Those with NCGS are negative for endomysial antibodies (EMA IgG and EMA IgA) and for another type of antibody common in those with CD. Tissue transglutaminase is an enzyme that repairs damage in the body. People with CD often make antibodies that attack tissue transglutaminase (tTG IgG and tTG IgA).

A medically prescribed diet is necessary for treatment of CD. At this time, doctors recommend that those with NCGS go on the diet simply for symptom control and comfort. Because there are so many people following the GFD and because most of these patients are self-diagnosed, it is almost impossible to determine the prevalence of NCGS, though it is estimated to be between 5% and 13% of the worldwide population.

The Gluten Intolerance Group published this helpful information to help us understand the differences between CD and NCGS:

	CD	NCGS
tTG-IgA, IgG antibodies	Positive	Negative
EMA IgA-IgG antibodies	Positive	Negative
Allergy testing positive	No	No
Damage to intestine	Yes	No
GFD beneficial	Yes	Yes

Much research has now been done to define CD and understand its effect on the body. Now, more research is needed to better understand NCGS, determine its physical impact, and establish the long-term benefits of a GFD.

Wheat Allergy

A wheat allergy can cause gastrointestinal symptoms but most likely results in the sudden onset of symptoms such as difficulty swallowing, rash, and shortness of breath after ingesting wheat, even a small amount. In severe cases, it can be life-threatening.

Irritable Bowel Syndrome

Another related disease is irritable bowel syndrome (IBS), affecting 40,000,000 people in the United States. CD and NCGS are often mistaken for IBS because the symptoms are similar, including abdominal pain and bloating. However, CD and NCGS improve on a GFD, and IBS does not. The positive response to the GFD is currently the only criteria used to distinguish CD and NCGS from IBS. Researchers still have to determine the relationship of these diseases and more specific criteria to diagnose them.

Gluten Sensitivity in Autism and Schizophrenia

Individuals with autism could also be under the spectrum of NCGS. Many parents of autistic children are focusing on a gluten-free/casein-free diet based on anecdotal evidence that it can change behavior in their children. There is some ongoing research about the correlation between autism and a family history of autoimmune diseases; however, there have been no significant decisions about this.

There has also been research on the correlation of gluten sensitivity and schizophrenia. A group of patients put on a GFD for two weeks had improved symptoms. Another study showed that those with schizophrenia have IgG and IgA gliadin antibodies. Gliadin is the protein found in wheat and it is these antibodies that attack the immune system causing the inflammatory process in the small intestine that destroys the villi. It will be interesting to follow these studies to see if the GFD has long-term benefits.

CHAPTER 2

Diagnosis and Treatment

Success is to be measured not so much by the position that one has reached in life as by the obstacles which he has overcome while trying to succeed.
—Booker T. Washington.

People with CD can suffer with symptoms for years before being diagnosed. The key to better health is automatically turned when a diagnosis is rendered. However, the key opens the door to a healthy lifestyle only if a gluten-free diet (GFD) is maintained. Adhering to the diet reduces the risk of complications.

The typical individual with CD may go to many doctors before being diagnosed. Sometimes it is necessary for a person suffering with abdominal bloating, pain, diarrhea, and/or constipation to rule out other diseases. Some of the problems that should be ruled out are irritable bowel syndrome (IBS), Crohn's disease, ulcerative colitis, diverticulitis, intestinal infection, chronic fatigue syndrome, and possibly other conditions not associated with the intestinal tract. The latest research shows that many who were diagnosed with IBS are being correctly diagnosed with CD.

The first step to a diagnosis begins with a laboratory test. *Continue to eat gluten until tested.* If you do not ingest gluten, the protein that causes the antibodies will not be present to indicate CD, even if you have it.

The panel usually done for the Celiac Profile is by the ELISA method (the enzyme-linked immunosorbent assay is a test that uses antibodies and color change to identify a substance) and includes:

Total IgA: 80% sensitive to CD
Tissue transglutaminase IgG and IgA (tTG IgG and tTG IgA): 95% sensitive to CD
Immunoflourescent Endomysial IgA (EMA IgA): 90% sensitive and 98% specific to CD

IgA, or the immunoglobulin A type of antibody, helps your body fight off common threats such as bacteria, viruses, and toxins. Research shows that people with CD are about ten to fifteen times more likely to have IgA deficiency than people without the condition.

If your total serum IgA test shows that you're IgA-deficient, that doesn't necessarily indicate you have CD. Common autoimmune conditions found with IgA deficiency include rheumatoid arthritis, lupus, and CD. If IgA is deficient, it is recommended that the deamidated gliadin peptide IgG (DGP IgG) and deamidated gliadin peptide IgA (DGP IgA) tests be ordered. The results of the DGP IgG, DGP IgA, and tTG IgA will allow for a differentiation between CD and an IgA deficiency.

It is very important to make sure that the laboratory doing the profile is familiar with this testing and, if in doubt, have it sent to a lab in a university setting with a CD center. The national laboratories most familiar with these profiles are Prometheus and Quest.

If your blood tests (tTG and EMA) are positive, it is recommended that your physician follow up with an endoscopy, in which a biopsy is done to identify the extent of damage to the small intestine. This test is done in an outpatient facility. It is recommended that six specimens be taken to make sure that enough areas are examined for diagnosis.

A flexible tube with a camera at the end is introduced through the stomach and into the small intestine. A mild sedative is usually given as part of this procedure. The endoscopy allows a gastroenterologist to examine the intestine and take a biopsy. The specimen is then sent to the laboratory to verify the diagnosis. The diagnosis of CD is made according to the Marsh Classifications from these biopsies. They are from type 0, type 1, type 2, type 3 and type 4. Type 0 is normal, type 1 shows increased infiltration of lymphocytes, type 2 shows crypt hyperplasia, type 3 shows blunting of the villi, and type 4 shows complete flattening.

A new technology for this examination is called the *wireless capsule endoscopy*. A miniaturized camera is swallowed and the remote camera visualizes the intestine. The problem with this procedure is that, if the villi are flat, then a regular endoscopy still must be done for the biopsy. It is anticipated that in the near future an endoscopy will not be necessary.

Genetics and CD. The individual must have a genetic predisposition to activate CD. According to Dr. Peter Green of Columbia University, 98% of people with CD share the genes identified as HLA-DQ2 and HLA-DQ8. He states that "People who do not have HLA-DQ2 or HLA-DQ8 haplotypes are unlikely to have coeliac disease." It is possible to have symptoms and, if a genetic test is run and these haplotypes are not present, still not fit the diagnosis of CD. One of the haplotypes of DQ2 or DQ8 must be present for CD.

There is discussion as to when the genetics test should be considered. People who might benefit:

* **People who are already on a GFD.** Unlike antibody tests and small intestine biopsies, DNA testing is accurate even when a person is already on a GFD. A positive test would increase the likelihood that their symptoms were caused by CD. A negative genetic test, however, would mean they do not have CD.
* **First-degree relatives of people with CD.** According to the University of Chicago Celiac Disease Center, if you are a first-degree relative (parent, child, or sibling) of a person with CD, you have a 1 in 22 chance of developing the disease in your lifetime. Statistics show that the immediate family members are also more prone to other autoimmune diseases.
* **People with unclear small bowel biopsy results.** If the results of the biopsy are not conclusive and the patient does not have either the DQ8 or DQ2 gene, then CD is unlikely.

Once the diagnosis is obtained, the challenge of managing the disease begins. Following a GFD for life is now the standard treatment. If gluten is ingested, the intestinal villi are destroyed. By eating gluten-free foods, the villi are not challenged or irritated by the gluten protein, and so are allowed to heal. This does take time. The first few months may cause some anxious moments if you think you've eaten something that contains gluten.

> CD is isolating, and the isolation can hurt far more than the treatment. Suddenly, you find yourself on one side of a fence, the sick side. Everyone else in your world is on the other side of that fence—the normal side.

After you begin the diet, it will take a few weeks, or even months, to start feeling an improvement in your health. It has been shown that the older the patient is at diagnosis, the longer that the villi take to heal. It has been found that sometimes they never completely heal on older patients. The amount of irritation CD has wrought on your body varies, as does the time required for the healing process. Do not be discouraged. Stay on the GFD.

If you are not feeling well and wondering why, you may have to re-evaluate your diet to make sure you're not eating anything—vitamin pills, candies, medicines, or foods—that may contain gluten. Read labels, read labels, read labels. Start a journal and write down everything that you eat. That is the best way to determine if you have accidentally ingested gluten.

There are some new "point of care" tests with both professional and at-home versions but the results of these should be read by a health care professional. Individuals should realize that the test may be inconclusive, may give a false negative, and is not meant for a final diagnosis.

Diagnosing Children

The criteria used to diagnosis adults cannot be used to diagnose children since the symptoms are so different at the onset. Many children go to their doctors with unrelated symptoms, such as growth failure, malabsorption, and unstable diabetes; many pediatricians now suggest that all type I diabetic children be screened for CD.

Children are less sensitive to the tTG test and pediatric gastroenterologists have found that DGP (deamidated gluten peptide) is more effective in diagnosing children.

Early Diagnosis Is Important

Take a proactive role in your child's health problems. Ask your physician to order the necessary tests to rule out other possibilities. The importance of physicians diagnosing CD within the early stages was discussed in an article published by Leffler, Saha, and Farrell in *The Managed Care Journal*.

It states that early diagnosis can prevent many of the complications associated with the disease, including osteoporosis and cancer. If you continue to have symptoms, and you've been unsuccessful in obtaining a clear diagnosis, take this book, a copy of your assessment, or a copy of the bibliography in the back of this book to your physician and ask him/her to consider the possibility that you may have CD.

For physicians as well as for patients, the learning curve at this juncture is difficult. Even though the amount of knowledge available is increasing, many health professionals are still unfamiliar with the disease. When this happens, you need to be persistent and show that you are an informed person who wants the answers to your questions. The more you know about CD, the easier it will be to make the adjustment to living a gluten-free lifestyle. Educating family and friends with adequate information will allow them to help you stay on the diet. Some family members may not understand your child's special dietary needs, and it may be necessary to take food with you when you visit, or invite them to sample a gluten-free meal. It may take months of educating, but eventually most people will understand that you must follow a very strict diet, and they will be glad to help you. It may be helpful if you can compare your dietary restrictions to those who have other diet-related disorders, such as diabetes or food allergies.

You can use the celiac iceberg (see Figure 2.1) to help explain the prevalence of the disease:

* The top one-third are the patients with symptoms and the gene who have been diagnosed with blood tests and biopsy.
* The middle third has silent CD. They have the gene but no symptoms, though they do have a "leaky gut" and damage to the small intestine.
* The bottom one-third (or more) is latent CD. They have the gene and have tested positive for antibodies but have a normal gut.

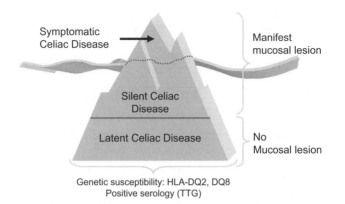

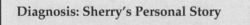

Genetic susceptibility: HLA-DQ2, DQ8
Positive serology (TTG)

Figure 2-1. The celiac iceberg.

The difficulty is that there is potential for long-term health problems for those undiagnosed. The genetic testing may be cost effective considering the prevention of the other conditions that are associated with undiagnosed CD.

Diagnosis: Sherry's Personal Story

"The symptom that eventually led my doctors to a diagnosis of celiac disease is not a classic symptom of the condition. The swallowing trouble I began having at age 39 was an atypical symptom and puzzled my doctors and me for four years. After several noninvasive tests that were negative for any causes of swallowing problems (e.g., cancer), my doctors concluded that anxiety might be the cause.

"Not convinced, I underwent both an endoscopy and esophageal manometry, which revealed the muscles were not functioning normally. The question that remained unanswered for the next 4 years was Why?

"After a few years of eating soft foods, which, ironically, were high gluten-containing foods like pasta, and taking antacids, I pressed my gastroenterologist for more testing.

(*continued*)

Diagnosis: Sherry's Personal Story (*continued*)

During the second endoscopy, a biopsy tested positive for *sprue* (which is another name for celiac disease). I will always remember my doctor saying, 'Don't worry,' and reassuring me that I could not possibly have this because it was too rare! But, because the test was positive, he ordered blood work, which confirmed the surprising diagnosis. I finally had some answers about why I was anemic, why I lost so much weight, and why I had trouble eating!

"Since CD was considered rare at the time (I was diagnosed in 1993), the first dietitian I went to admitted that she would have to learn along with me. Luckily, she had some familiarity with gluten-free foods to recommend to me, and she also sent for diet information from the Gluten Intolerance Group of America.

"After months of struggling to make sense of all the new and sometimes conflicting information about the diet, I learned about our support group in Columbus. I was excited to learn about the annual celiac conferences organized by clinical dietitian, Mary Kay Sharrett and Dr. B. Li of Children's Hospital, both of whom had special interests in supporting and educating celiac patients. What a relief it was to get the guidance I needed to follow a GF diet, and support others with CD, to help me meet all the challenges that sometimes seemed overwhelming."

Diagnosis: A Member of the Gluten-Free Gang Support Group's Personal Story

"I had crunched ice most of my life, but never like this. When I was pregnant with my second child, I would go through the ice from our automatic icemaker so fast that I bought four extra ice cube trays to freeze each day to keep up with my 'demand.' When that supply was exhausted, I would beg my husband to go buy me a 10-pound bag of ice. This was a sign of anemia caused by my undiagnosed

(*continued*)

celiac disease. I was severely anemic, experiencing extreme fatigue, heart palpitations, and shortness of breath. I had no gastrointestinal symptoms or weight loss. My due date was approaching and, to ensure a safe delivery, I was given a blood transfusion and multiple intravenous iron infusions. In the end, the doctors (my OBGYN and hematologist) concluded that the anemia had been caused by the pregnancy.

"About one month after the baby was born, I suddenly began having severe diarrhea. At first, I assumed that I had eaten a bad hamburger at a fast food restaurant the day before it started. However, the diarrhea would not go away. I called my doctor who, after informing me that viruses were going around, prescribed an antidiarrheal medication. It did help a little bit with the symptoms, but I was still afraid to leave my house (and my bathroom). After complaining to the doctor a few more times, he decided to test my stool for infectious organisms. The results were negative.

"I had a feeling that my problems were due to more than just a virus. I called the doctor one more time, and he did the best thing he could have done. He referred me to a gastroenterologist. After a colonoscopy, an upper endoscopy, and a simple blood test, it was confirmed that I had celiac sprue disease, five months after my initial bout with diarrhea had appeared.

"I have been on the gluten-free diet for a little over a year, and I am happy to say that the ice cubes in my freezer are going stale for the first time that I can ever remember."

Living with CD

The best way to start treating your CD is to ask for a care conference (see Figure 2.2) that includes your doctor, dietitian, family, pharmacist, registered nurse, and a member of a CD support group. This is the ideal way to obtain valuable information, provide the best continuity of care, and

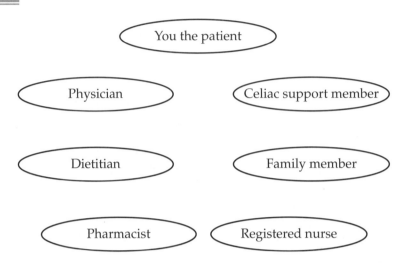

Figure 2-2. Care conference.

achieve the best optimum outcome. Within the medical profession, many complicated problems are approached using this method, so you are justified in asking for this.

The professionals participating in a care conference represent different disciplines. Each will present information about his/her particular aspect of the disease and how it affects you. Your general physician will be aware of your total medical condition, prescription medications you are taking, and the results of the testing that you have had, and he may wish to share a plan for specific follow up. Your dietitian will be able to make recommendations for dietary changes and offer resources regarding food supply and educational opportunities. A registered nurse may be asked to coordinate all disciplines, acting as your patient advocate, and to assist in creating a plan of care for you. Your family members will gain a better understanding of the challenges, genetic predisposition, common symptoms, and the necessity of a lifelong diet in CD. Finally, your pharmacist can evaluate all your medications to see if they contain gluten. Your individual needs can be best met through this multidisciplinary approach. It is the most effective way for all disciplines to understand what approach will work best to get you on the road to recovery. If you cannot assemble a care team in one room, then speak with them individually. It is most important to meet with a dietitian familiar with CD to determine the list of foods allowed and where to obtain them.

Remember, being in charge of your diet is the most important thing you can do. You still have all your strengths and abilities. The disease has nothing to do with that. By taking control, you can remain confident and have the assurance of living a healthy life. Sherry summarized her story with a remarkable ending. "The GF diet consists of many healthy foods and includes a surprising variety of alternative grains. I am grateful to have answers to many life-long problems and thankful that I have a condition that can be treated through dietary modification. What continues to motivate me is the commitment to better health and desire to set a good example for my adult children."

It is my prayer that the content of this book and the many other resources mentioned, will enable you to have a positive and healthy outlook on your CD. Embrace it and find the real you in it!

Living with CD: Forrest's Personal Story

"In 1990, when I was two years old my parents noticed a decrease in my energy level and that my belly was getting larger and larger. My father took me to the emergency room because of the abrupt change in my condition.

"The hospital couldn't figure out what was going on. They kept giving me tests, but no answers were coming. They even had me quarantined in the ER for a while to see if it was contagious. After being admitted and still no answers they were talking about doing exploratory surgery

---

(continued)

Living with CD: Forrest's Personal Story (*continued*)

to see what was going on. They even had an adrenaline shot taped to my chart, just in case they needed it. Finally a pediatric gastroenterologist saw my extreme malnutrition, looked at my cuticles, and teeth, and asked about our heritage (Irish and English). She ordered a biopsy to look at my small intestines, and that is when they realized that I had CD.

"At that time the medical community thought that 1 out of 2,000 adults had it and only 1 out of 60,000 children could have it. There was very little known about CD at this time, so I became a very popular patient in the hospital. One day the hospital dietitian walked into my room and found the nurse feeding me a Boston cream pie. She had just taken the top off of it so she could feed me the cream out of the center because it did not have gluten in it. At that point, the dietitian told my parents that they needed to take me and feed me bacon and eggs for breakfast and plain meat and potatoes for other meals. She said that if they kept me on this kind of diet for two weeks, they would have a new child with all kinds of energy again.

Going through the cupboards at home to remove all the items that could possibly have any gluten in them was an eye-opening experience for my parents. Most of the food in the pantry contained gluten, so quick, easy convenience foods were no longer an option for our family. My parents started looking at other gluten-free food options. They soon realized that a simple trip to the grocery store could take up to two hours. They had to read every label, write down the phone number of each manufacturer, and then go home and call to find out what the product's 'modified food starch' was or if some other ingredient might contain gluten. This took place every time we went to the store.

"My parents would buy me gluten-free bread and be very insistent that I was going to eat it all, because they spent over six dollars on it. The problem was that this

Living with CD: Forrest's Personal Story (*continued*)

bread could be thrown across the room, hit the wall, and not break. And that was the major part of every one of my sandwiches! A lot has changed since then. The food has gotten better, more people are realizing that they can't have gluten, and we don't have to call the manufacturers of every food product anymore.

"As I grew up with CD, I was always looking for new food options. Around the time I started high school, information about oats being gluten free as long as they were from a pure source and not cross-contaminated was coming out. I had never had an oatmeal cookie or bowl of oatmeal before so I decided to try and come up with a way to offer 'safe' oats. That was the beginning of my business, GF Harvest (www.glutenfreeoats.com), that sells oatmeal and dozens of other gluten-free products. In my family, we have 10 members that are diagnosed with CD. Both of my parents have found out that they have it, and my sister has the gene but not the symptoms yet. We understand what it means to live your life as a celiac and take the threat of cross-contamination seriously.

"Yes, I have to say that parts of life have been hard for me and my family but at the same time being diagnosed with CD at such a young age was really a giant blessing. It has allowed me to be part of the gluten-free community, see it grow, and be part of a new food option for all of us on a GFD.

"No matter how discouraged you become, try to recognize that this is not a problem but an opportunity, and move forward to the next good thing coming."

CHAPTER 3

Dermatitis Herpetiformis

Life is a pure flame, and we live by an invisible sun within us.

—Thomas Browne

Dermatitis herpetiformis (DH) is a chronic eruption of the skin characterized by clusters of intensely itchy, small bubbles and allergy- or hive-like lesions that are slow to heal (Figure 3-1). The disease is usually found in patients 30 to 40 years old and is more common in men than in women. It occurs rarely in African Americans and Asians. All normal appearing skin will have antibody (IgA) deposits. The rash, which is caused by an allergic reaction to gluten, is called "celiac disease of the skin."

The herpes virus does not cause DH, even though the name suggests it. Herpetiformis means "grouped vessels" and describes the rash that accompanies DH. The rash is often confused with other kinds of allergic skin rashes. As mentioned above, the actual cause is the body's response to the gluten protein found in wheat, barley, and rye. Allergies like hives are usually caused by the IgE antibodies of the immune system. DH is caused by the IgA antibody, which is produced in the lining of

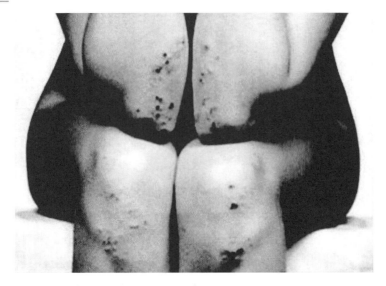

Figure 3-1. An example of dermatitis herpetiformis. (Used with permission from the University of Chicago Celiac Research Center.)

the intestine. The usual forms of allergy treatments are not effective in treating DH.

When the gut is affected by the inflammatory response to the proteins in wheat, barley, and rye so that the villi are inflamed and/or destroyed, it is called gluten-sensitive enteropathy (GSE), or celiac disease (CD). Some people with DH do not have GSE and others do. Because there are cases of GSE that have turned cancerous (malignant lymphoma), an evaluation by a gastroenterologist is important. It is interesting that the signs and symptoms of malabsorption in DH are usually absent, and there is no association between the intensity of the intestinal damage found at biopsy of the small intestine and the intensity of the skin lesions in DH. CD is found in 75% to 90% of DH patients, indicating that they are directly connected to CD.

Dr. Stefano Guandalini from the University of Chicago Celiac Disease Program wrote an article for the *DX: Celiac* newsletter which he has agreed to allow us to include here. The article is one of the most recent and comprehensive statements about DH, and the authors thank him for his permission to use it.

Dermatitis herpetiformis (DH) is a condition that raises many questions and concerns among parents and patients, ranging from how to distinguish an allergic skin reaction from actual DH to the optimal management of DH once diagnosed.

DH is an uncommon skin manifestation of CD, affecting mostly adults. It has a prevalence of approximately one to two in 10,000 people. DH is characterized by the appearance of small pimples and blisters, typically on the elbows. They may also appear on the knees, face, scalp, trunk, buttocks, and occasionally within the mouth. The lesions are symmetrically diffused. The predominant symptoms are itching and burning that is rapidly relieved when the blisters rupture.

The earliest abnormality is a small reddish spot about one-eighth of an inch in diameter that quickly develops into a "bump." Small blisters then appear and tend to merge together. Scratching causes them to rupture, dry up, and leave an area of darker color and scarring.

As DH is not common, usually the diagnosis takes a long time. The dermatologist will confirm DH by obtaining a skin biopsy (best if taken at the edge of the lesion, not on the affected skin). The pathology exam of the biopsy will show the typical deposition of granular immunoglobulin A (IgA) in the skin by a microscopic exam with a method called immunofluorescence. The disease is in fact thought to result from an aggression of IgA auto antibodies directed against the skin-associated tissue transglutaminase.

What makes DH unique is its association with CD. In fact, DH is celiac disease: they share exactly the same genetic background (DQ2 and/or DQ8), each condition is more frequent in families where the other is also found, they are both triggered by an autoimmune response to gluten, and they are associated with other autoimmune conditions such as thyroiditis (found in as many as one in four DH patients.)

DH and CD also are characterized by the same type of gluten-induced damage to the intestinal mucosa (the flattening of the villi) and they both carry an increased risk—when not treated—of lymphomas.

Thus, if DH is diagnosed, celiac disease is also present and the same strict gluten-free diet must be started.

Dr. Guandalini also describes the differences between DH and CD:

* The predominance of females vs. males in CD is reversed: DH is found twice as frequently in males.
* The mean age of onset is later in DH, around 40 years, with childhood DH being a rare occurrence.
* There is a higher prevalence (about 20%) of serologically negative (tissue transglutaminase and/or endomysial antibodies negative) patients with DH; therefore serological screening in DH is not as effective as it is in celiac disease.
* Signs and symptoms of malabsorption in DH are usually absent or minor.
* There is no association between the intensity of the intestinal damage found at biopsy of the small intestine and the intensity of the skin lesions in DH.

He goes on to say:

Because of the typical gastrointestinal problems and the slow response (months to years) to a strict gluten-free diet (GFD), some patients with DH think they have no benefit from the diet and do not follow it, relying only on the pharmacological treatment with Dapsone. *This is a mistake!* Dapsone will suppress, but not cure the disease, and is completely ineffective on the intestinal lesion: on the other hand, GFD results in clearing of the skin disease and of the intestinal damage. To further support this concept, reintroduction of gluten has been found to result in the recurrence of the disease (within weeks).

Correctly treating this disorder and preventing its complications, requires the daily use of oral Dapsone (that relieves the itching within two days) and an ongoing, strict GFD. Dapsone is tapered off as time on the gluten-free diet lengthens, and Dapsone should eventually be discontinued.

Continuing on a strict GFD is still considered the best treatment for CD and DH. Both conditions are genetic and both cause destruction in the small intestine. According to an article reviewing DH in 2013, the HLA DQ2 genotype is found in 80% to 90% of cases. For the individual with DH a GFD will help control symptoms, decrease small intestinal damage, decrease risk of lymphoma, and improve quality of life. The frustration that occurs with DH is that it can take a long time for the lesions to clear after going gluten free (GF). Those patients with DH treated with a GFD and Dapsone can still show increased risk of osteoporosis due to the lack of absorption of calcium in the small intestine. Autoimmune diseases, such as thyroid (5%–11%), pernicious anemia (1%–3%), type 1 diabetes (1%–2%), and collagen tissue disease, also present at higher levels in those with DH.

There has always been a question as to whether topical items such as shampoo, lotions, and other skin products need to be GF for the celiac. Dr. Peter Green in his book *Celiac Disease: A Hidden Epidemic* states "that unless you are eating these products, they are not going to cause a DH flare-up."

Bob, a professional man, came to the Gluten-Free Gang, a celiac disease support group, when he was first diagnosed with DH. He agreed to give us his story and experiences with DH.

It was not long after I developed a very itchy rash on my elbows, forearms, knees, and sacrum in late 2000 that I made an appointment with a dermatologist to have it checked out. The itch was so intense it pretty much consumed my everyday life and was more severe than I was accustomed to experiencing with poison ivy on numerous occasions throughout my life. Attempts at using topical creams to alleviate the itch were, for the most part, futile. I probably suffered through it for about three months until I sought medical help. Although the first dermatologist noted I exhibited the classic findings of DH, the initial skin biopsy proved to be taken improperly, which resulted in negative immunofluorescense results. A follow-up punch biopsy by another dermatologist a few months later proved to be successful and I was clinically diagnosed with DH.

During the interim between both biopsies, I was prescribed Dapsone to see if it would alleviate the rash. It literally only took about two to three hours for the intense itching to completely subside. Although the rash was still present and took longer to somewhat clear up, it was a relief the itch abated and I was able to get a full night's sleep. The dermatologist mentioned I was probably only the second case of DH he's ever diagnosed and that the disease was due to having wheat in my diet. That's all I was told as I walked out his door.

I had no idea what the rash really entailed until I researched it on my own through Internet searches and discovered it was closely associated with an incurable condition called celiac disease and that the only lifetime treatment for it was the adherence to a GFD. Unlike a classic celiac patient, I had no gastrointestinal symptoms such as cramping, diarrhea, or constipation. The only indication that I suffered intestinal damage was a history (at least five years) of anemia. I also learned that some environmental/stressful factor or body trauma likely triggers the disease to begin manifesting itself. In my case, it may have been attributed to a surgery I had in July 1998.

I was pretty overwhelmed after learning all the foods I was no longer able to eat. At the time of my diagnosis, I was 30 years old, athletic, and very active. I had (and still maintain) a high metabolism and was always eating. I relied heavily on carbohydrates, particularly for breakfast and snacks. I realized I needed some counseling to help me with the dietary change. To just suddenly give up certain foods, particularly breads, desserts, pasta, and beer was quite a sacrifice—especially my mom's Hungarian cooking and pastries! Through the Internet, I contacted the Gluten Intolerance Group in Seattle, and was referred to a Central Ohio dietitian, Mary Kay Sharrett, who dealt closely with celiac patients and served as a liaison for a local support group called the Gluten-Free Gang. My initial anxiety about trying to adhere to a GFD was alleviated after I met with Mary Kay for diet instruction and began attending the group meetings for tips and guidance.

Through time, I gradually adjusted to the change in my diet and was able to adapt by substituting certain foods for what I used to consume. I had to learn to accept that I might never be able to taste the foods I grew up with my entire life—there was no turning back. I have to admit, I am a pretty dedicated person and will stick to a regimen if it is for my well-being. I was never a finicky eater. I ate just about anything, anytime, that was put in front of me. I was challenged all the time, particularly when I had to leave my comfort zone at home and travel for work, typically every six weeks, most of the time to San Diego or the San Francisco Bay areas. I was lucky in this respect and couldn't have asked for better destinations. California was famous for its abundance of health-food stores and seafood and Mexican cuisines. However, I also traveled to remote places in West Virginia as well as in the Deep South, where just about everything is fried. No matter where my travels took me, once arriving at my destination, I would immediately go grocery shopping, particularly for breakfast and lunch items. I always stayed in hotel rooms equipped with a fridge and microwave at a minimum. If small kitchens were available, I requested those rooms. During the workday, I always packed my lunch and abundant snacks in a small cooler. On numerous occasions when eating out with co-workers when we were travelling, I would usually agree to the consensus of where to eat without knowing the menu. It was too embarrassing and complicated trying to explain my restricted diet to everyone, and there was no way I was going to rain on their parade with the wide choice of cuisines that San Diego and the Bay Area offered. Because I was not a finicky eater, there was always something I could eat, even if it meant having just a salad at an Italian restaurant to hold me over until I got back to my stash in the hotel room. With time, my close friends and coworkers became understanding of my diet and were willing at times to compromise their choice of cuisine for my sake.

At home, my wife was also trying to deal with the dietary change. I would usually kid her that it was pretty coincidental that my DH/CD manifested soon after we got married. I never expected her to surrender her diet to accommodate mine. In actuality, I only had to tailor my diet slightly to adapt to what we made in the past. We always maintained a healthy diet. We rarely ate fast food, frozen dinners, or prepared fried foods. I had my own cupboard with my own pastas, flours, mixes, etc. I picked up on a good sourdough recipe for bread through the Gluten-Free Gang and bake my own buns for sandwiches. The only specialty foods I purchase from health food stores are GF cereals, pancake mixes, pastas, crackers, and the occasional brownie mix. I really never had a sweet tooth so only once in a blue moon do I buy GF cookies and cakes.

However, I was still coping with the rash flare-ups associated with DH. Even though I started omitting gluten from my diet, there was still an abundance of antibodies in my body from all the gluten I ingested in the past. I learned that it commonly took five to seven years until the body was rid of the antibodies that caused the skin disorder. Wow, I thought—seven years of an intense constant itch that I had to try to maintain with the Dapsone. Even though the Dapsone alleviated the itch most of the time, the rash would still erupt spontaneously, resulting in constant scratching that opened sores and caused them to bleed, soiling my clothes, our linens, furniture, etc. After the sores scabbed up, they, too, warranted scratching because they were typically located on joints that were subjected to constant stretching and irritation. It was embarrassing in public because there was no way I could not scratch some part of my body, which usually led to bleeding. If I had a penny for every time my wife chastised me for scratching in public, I would have more than enough money to buy those heavily priced GF beers by the case. She just assumed I popped a pill (Dapsone) and my troubles would be over.

As the years went on, I had blood tests performed quarterly to determine, first, whether my antibody count was decreasing, and second, to make sure the Dapsone was not damaging my liver, thus enabling me to get refills. The serological testing was the only way I could gauge whether my diet was working. If I accidentally ingested gluten, which I have done at times on the GF diet, there was no way of knowing it. I was still getting the rash no matter what. With no rhyme or reason, the rash seemed to make it to just about every part of my body at some point.

Looking back, it is almost as if it would erupt pretty fiercely for six months to a year at one location before phasing out and going on to another body part. The rash would eventually develop on my scalp and the back of my neck (resulting in embarrassing trips to the barber), my eyebrows, underarms, elbows, forearms, wrists, scapula (most difficult part to scratch), hips, sacrum, buttocks, knees, calves, shins, and currently on my ankles and feet. Many times I wished I had the gastrointestinal symptoms because at least they manifested very soon after a mishap and I could deduce what foods I [had] consumed had gluten. Then I got to thinking: If I screwed up and accidentally ingested gluten at some point during the diet, did that seven-year clock reset itself from that point on? It was a very frustrating time. I tried to limit the dosage of Dapsone I took and only increased it when a rash erupted. Gradually, to my relief, the diet began to kick in, enabling me to decrease my dosage. Serological tests showed non detectable levels of antibodies. My rashes were not really erupting anymore but rather coming on slowly with minimal itching sensations.

Currently, after six years, I would have to say my body is about 95% GF. I do not think I will ever reach 100%, but it is to a stage where I am no longer taking Dapsone, but rather have it handy in case of an "episode." I never travel without it. I have learned that because my body is pretty much free of antibodies, when I do accidentally ingest gluten, it takes about ten days to two weeks for the rash to erupt (but who knows where on my body it will decide to show up) and last only about a month or two before clearing up. I still have minor rashes, but nothing compared to a full-blown eruption that would have me popping a Dapsone.

As a result of having full-blown DH for six years, I have developed a scratching habit, whether it is warranted or not, and almost as a nervous habit. My body is riddled with scars from constantly scratching the same scabs off numerous times, and (to my wife's relief) I am not doing laundry as much as I used to. Finally, I have to say that, at 38 years old, I am in the best health I have ever been.

A very honest testimony from Bob, who has been through it.

CHAPTER 4

A Healthy Gluten-Free Diet

Mary Kay Sharrett

We shall steer safely through every storm, so long as our heart is right, our intention fervent, our courage steadfast, and our trust fixed on God.

—St. Francis De Sales

A gluten-free diet (GFD) is the only treatment for celiac disease (CD). Therefore, making sure your food is gluten free (GF) is the key to staying healthy when you have CD. However, there are a few other actions you should take to make sure your diet is both GF *and* healthy.

At diagnosis, your body may be deficient in several nutrients because gluten damaged your small intestine. The GFD can be low in B vitamins, iron, calcium, and fiber for two reasons. First, most GF grain products are not enriched or fortified with B vitamins and iron, as their gluten-containing counterparts are required to be. In addition, many GF grain products are based on corn, potato, and rice starches which have been stripped of fiber and other nutrients. Some people with CD have trouble tolerating milk and they have decreased or eliminated milk and milk products from their diets, thus making their diets deficient in calcium, vitamin D, and vitamin B_1. GF baked goods including bread, bagels, pretzels, cake, doughnuts, and cookies can contain significantly more fat and sugar than those with gluten. As you can see, it is not only important to learn what foods are GF, but also to learn what foods to include in your diet to stay healthy.

Making It Gluten Free

The first step in living with CD is learning what foods are GF. The GFD eliminates all foods prepared with wheat, rye, barley, and any ingredient made from these grains or any food or ingredient that comes in contact with them. Several recent studies have indicated that oats, in moderate amounts (½ cup), is safe for the majority of adults and children with CD. However, the cross-contamination of oats with other gluten-containing grains during the harvesting and milling process is a concern. Therefore, oats need to be specially handled from the field to the final product and they need to say "gluten free" on the label to be considered safe.

The following grains and/or starches are naturally GF:

Amaranth	Millet
Arrowroot	Nuts
Bean	Potato
Bean flour	Quinoa
Buckwheat	Rice
Corn	Sago
Flax	Sorghum hum
Indian rice grass	Soy
Legumes	Tapioca
Lentils	Teff
Mesquite	Wild rice

However, all these grains and starches can become contaminated during the milling and manufacturing process, so it is important to purchase them from manufacturers who take precautions to eliminate cross-contamination. Use only those that say "gluten free" on the label.

Reading Food Labels

All food labels must be carefully examined to determine product contents. (Table 4-1 lists ingredients to avoid.) Gluten can be in almost anything you put in your mouth. Medications may contain gluten (see Chapter 12). Prescription and over-the-counter medications need to be checked for gluten content.

Become an avid label reader. Food manufacturers do change their ingredients so make sure you read the label each time you purchase an item and then double check the labels before you prepare the food.

The Food Allergen Consumer Protection Act (FALCPA) (Public Law 108–282) was passed in the summer of 2004 and went into effect in January 2006. This law requires food manufacturers to declare the source of ingredients when they contain one of the top eight allergens (milk, eggs, peanuts, tree nuts, fish, crustacean shellfish, soy, and wheat). The allergen needs to be declared in plain language, meaning that if it is made from wheat it must declare *wheat* on the label. Oats, barley, and rye are not considered one of the top eight allergens However, oats and rye are not hidden in any ingredients. Barley is listed as barley, malt, or brewer's yeast. The likelihood that barley is hidden is extremely low. Therefore, you can read the label and look for the six words listed in Table 4-1 to determine if a product is GF.

There is an exception to the FALCPA allergen labeling laws, which apply to all foods governed by the FDA. The United States Department of Agriculture (USDA) governs

Table 4-1. Ingredients to avoid on a GFD

Look for the following 6 words on the label

* Wheat
* Rye
* Untested oats
* Barley
* Malt
* Brewer's yeast

meat, poultry, and eggs, and these products do not need to follow FALCPA. The good news is that the USDA says that 80% to 90% of the companies are following FALCPA. However, that still means that there may be some hidden wheat in the form of modified food starch, starch, or dextrin in some products.

Fresh meat, fresh poultry, and fresh eggs (in the shell) are not an issue. To determine if a processed product is governed by the USDA, check for a seal that says inspected by the USDA on the front of the package. For example, lunchmeat, hot dogs, sausage, liquid eggs, canned soups, and frozen dinners will fall into this category. If the label says "gluten free," then it is GF. If the product does not say "gluten free" and there is modified food starch, starch, or dextrin on the label, look to see if the product has a "contains" statement. If there is a "contains" statement such as "contains soy" and it does not say "contains wheat" or any of the other six gluten-containing ingredients, then it is safe because if they declared one allergen, they would have declared all of them, including wheat. If you see that there is no "contains" statement, check with the manufacturer about the source of these ingredients.

FALCPA also directed the FDA to define the term gluten free. The FDA released the final definition in August 2013. When you find the words "gluten free" on a label, it means that the food contains less than 20 parts per million (ppm) of the protein gluten. There are several studies that show that most people with CD can tolerate trace amounts of gluten in foods. The level of less than 20 ppm was used by the FDA because it did a safety assessment and found that it is the lowest level that can be reliably tested in all foods. Less than 20 ppm is also consistent with the levels other countries use to define GF.

U.S. Food and Drug Administration Labeling Laws

According to the FDA Labeling rules in effect as of August 5, 2014, to be labeled "gluten free" a product must have less than 20 ppm of gluten from wheat, barley, or rye. This includes goods that are imported into the United States and dietary supplements.

Not covered:

* Foods under U.S. Department of Agriculture's jurisdiction (USDA) including meat, poultry, and certain egg products.
* Foods under the jurisdiction of the Alcohol and Tobacco Tax and Trade Bureau (TTB), including distilled spirits or wines with 7% or more alcohol by volume and malted beverages made with malted barley and hops.

The FDA will be working with both the USDA and the TTB to harmonize their respective labeling requirements.

Other key facts of the law:

* Food manufacturers will not be required to test their products, however, they are responsible for ensuring that the food product meets all labeling requirements.
* The rule is voluntary. A manufacturer may opt-out of labeling a product GF even if it does not contain gluten and complies with the labeling rule.
* A label that reads "no gluten," "free of gluten," or "without gluten" will be interpreted to mean "gluten free."
* It is unclear how the new regulation will affect restaurants that make GF claims on their menus.

Make It Nutritious

A healthy GFD should include a wide variety of foods. For the majority of adults and children, your diet should include two to four servings of fruits, three to five servings of vegetables, six to eleven servings of GF grains, and three to four servings from the milk food group. Making wise choices from all of these food groups can help provide the nutrients that are of concern in the GFD. Check out www .choosemyplate.gov to help you determine serving sizes and tailor these recommendations to meet your needs. There are several GF grains included in the whole grain section.

Enriched? Fortified?

Enriched and fortified mean that a food has nutrients (usually vitamins and minerals) added to it to make it more nutritious. *Enriched* is defined as adding back nutrients that were lost during the processing of the product. *Fortified* means adding nutrients to a product that are not present in the original product. In the 1940s, the U.S. FDA developed standards for refined white flour. Their original goal was to add the thiamine, niacin, and riboflavin (the B vitamins) lost during the processing of wheat. Since then, the FDA has required the addition of iron and folic acid. They have also made provisions for the optional addition of calcium. These standards were developed because of concern that American diets were deficient in these nutrients. GF grain products are not required to be enriched and fortified. However, many foods allowable in the GFD, especially GF whole grains, fruits, vegetables, nuts, seeds and legumes, are good sources of these nutrients (Table 4-2). There are some enriched and fortified GF products available, especially in the cereal aisle.

Fiber

The Dietary Reference Intakes (DRIs) recommend that Americans increase their intake of fiber because it can help prevent and treat many different health-related issues such as obesity, cardiovascular disease, type 2 diabetes, and constipation. The DRI for children 1 to 3 years old is 19 grams of fiber per day; for children 4 to 6 years old, 25 grams per day; for teenage boys, 31 grams; for teenage girls, 26 grams; for men age 19 to 50 years, 38 grams, and age 51 and older, 31 grams; for women 19 to 50 years, 25 grams, and age 51 and older, 21 grams. Yet the average American only eats 11 grams of fiber per day.

Constipation, rising cholesterol levels, and weight control problems are common issues among CD patients following a GFD. (See Table 4-3 for high fiber intake.) You can find out how much fiber is in your diet by looking at the Nutrient Facts Label on your food. Remember to look at the serving size, too. If you are not eating enough fiber, gradually add more to your diet—but do it slowly, because

Table 4-2. Some food sources of nutrients

Iron	Folate	Thiamin
Best sources: Pork loin, sardines, molasses, oysters, clams. *Good sources:* Lean beef, kidney beans, amaranth spinach, shrimp, pinto beans, greens, tuna, navy beans, avocado, dried apricots, tempeh (soy product), lentils, raisins, potatoes with skin, green peas, lima beans, prunes, figs	Liver and other organ meats, eggs, spinach, pineapple, tomato juice, asparagus, corn, bananas, amaranth, millet, teff, wild rice, enriched GF cereals	*Good sources:* Beef liver, pork (lean), millet, teff, enriched corn tortilla, enriched corn grits, enriched rice, brown rice, enriched GF cereals. *Fair sources:* Cantaloupe, honeydew, orange juice, watermelon, corn, peas, dry beans, lentils, pine nuts, sunflower seeds, peanuts

(continued)

Table 4-2. Some food sources of nutrients (*continued*)

Riboflavin	Niacin	Vitamin B$_{12}$
Good sources: Beef liver, yogurt, milk, enriched corn tortilla, egg, millet, quinoa, wild rice, enriched GF cereals. *Fair sources:* Broccoli, mushrooms, spinach, sweet potato, almonds	*Good sources:* Turkey, peanut butter, enriched corn tortilla, codfish, black-eyed peas, lima beans, wild rice, buckwheat, brown rice, millet, enriched cereals	Organ meats (beef and lamb liver, kidney, heart), clams, oysters, nonfat dry milk, crabs, salmon, sardines, rock fish, egg yolk

Table 4-3. Tips for increasing your fiber intake

* Add kidney beans, garbanzos, or other bean varieties into your salads. Each half-cup serving contains approximately 7 to 8 grams of fiber.
* Use whole-grain flour when possible in your cooking and baking, and choose whole-grain bread. Some GF flours that are high in fiber are buckwheat, amaranth, quinoa, corn meal, garbanzo flour (chickpea), garfava flour (garbanzo and fava beans).
* GF whole grains like quinoa make great side dishes or can be added to soups, stews, and other side or main dishes.
* Eat at least five servings each day of fruits and vegetables. Juices don't have fiber. Fresh fruit has slightly higher fiber content than canned. While all fruits have some fiber, some are higher than others. A few that have 3 to 4 grams of fiber per serving include apples, pears, 1 cup of blueberries, 1 cup of strawberries, oranges, and tangerines. Raspberries are high in fiber, with 8 grams per cup. Vegetables can be good sources of fiber also. Those that have 3 to 4 grams of fiber include: ½-cup squash, ½-cup peas, 1 cup carrots, ½-cup cauliflower, and 1 medium sweet potato.

(continued)

Table 4-3. Tips for increasing your fiber intake (*continued*)

---

* Add chopped dried fruits to your cookies, muffins, pancakes, or breads before baking. Dried fruits have a higher amount of fiber than the fresh version. For example, 1 cup of grapes has about 1 gram of fiber, but 1 cup of raisins has almost 7 grams. Packaged fruit leathers or snacks have no fiber.
* Nuts and seeds are excellent sources of fiber (avoid offering to children under age 4 who may choke on these). A ¼ cup of the following nuts and seeds contain 3 to 4 grams of fiber: sunflower seeds, peanuts, sesame seeds, and almonds.
* Add flax. Flax is a great source of fiber and other nutrients. Flax seed must be broken up in order for you to absorb nutrients and benefit from the fiber Use a coffee grinder to grind the seed, and grind as you need it. You can store whole flax seed at room temperature. Store ground flax in the refrigerator or freezer. Add it to cereals and yogurts.
* Cook with brown rice rather than white rice. If it's hard to make the switch, mix them together. One cup of brown rice is 3½ grams of fiber. Wild rice is also a good source of fiber—1 cup has 9 grams of fiber.
* Choose fiber-rich snacks such as popcorn (1 gram of fiber per cup), raw vegetables with reduced-fat dip, rice bran or flax seed crackers with cheese, and trail mix.

---

a large increase in your fiber intake at one time may cause you some abdominal discomfort and gas.

Lactose Intolerance

Lactose is the natural sugar found in milk. *Lactase* is the enzyme that digests lactose, and it is found on the tips of the villi in the small intestine. If your intestinal villi are damaged, then you may not be producing enough lactase. When lactose is undigested, it travels through the intestine and gets digested and used by the normal bacteria that reside there. This bacterial activity can cause gas and pain; it also attracts water to the intestine and usually results in diarrhea. Thirty to sixty percent of adults diagnosed with CD also have lactose intolerance. Very few children have lactose intolerance at diagnosis.

The treatment for lactose intolerance in conjunction with CD is a GFD and a temporary reduced-lactose diet. Once your intestine heals, you should be able to tolerate lactose, although some may never able to tolerate lactose. If you need to follow a lactose-restricted diet, you should eliminate milk and products made with milk such as ice cream, cottage cheese, and some other cheeses. However, these foods provide you with calcium and vitamin D, which are very important to your bone health. Many adults and children have low bone mineral density or even osteoporosis at diagnosis because they have not been absorbing calcium and vitamin D very well. Therefore, to maintain bone health, adequate intakes of calcium and vitamin D are important for newly diagnosed CD patients, as well as for everyone with CD.

If you have lactose intolerance, try to include milk that has been treated with an enzyme such as Lactaid. Aged cheese has very little lactose in it, and yogurt with active enzyme is usually well tolerated. You can also take an enzyme with your meals that will break down the lactose before it reaches the small intestine. Another tip is to eat lactose-containing foods with a meal, rather than between meals. If you still cannot tolerate three to four servings from the milk group, make sure you work with your dietitian to get the proper amounts of calcium and vitamin D supplements (GF supplements are listed on the website www .glutenfreedrugs.com).

Vitamins and Minerals

An age-appropriate multivitamin with minerals is recommended for people with CD. However, taking a multivitamin is not a substitute for good eating habits. Food provides an ideal mixture of essential nutrients that cannot be captured in a pill. Therefore, taking recommended amounts of vitamins and eating a healthy diet is recommended. Taking large doses of some vitamins or minerals can cause deficiencies of other vitamins or minerals, so be sure to work with your dietitian and doctor if you are taking more than the recommended amounts of vitamins and minerals. (GF vitamins and minerals can be found listed at www.glutenfree-drugs.com)

Read and learn as much as you can about CD and the GFD as well as about nutrition. You will soon find out that successfully following the GFD is less about what you need to take out of your diet and more about what you can add to it.

CHAPTER 5

Complications

The world will never starve for want of wonders.
—Gilbert Keith Chesterton

Most research recognizes celiac disease (CD) as a multisystem disorder. This means that it can have an effect on many different body systems. It was originally thought that the only organ involved in CD was the small intestine. It is now known that tissue transglutaminase antibody, commonly found in those with CD, is present in the gut, skin, and brain. This certainly verifies that CD is systemic, meaning it affects multiple systems in the body, and a number of other conditions have been found to be associated with CD. For example, researchers at Cornell University and the Minneapolis VA Hospital have recognized that neuropathy and several other neurologic syndromes are associated with CD, and that these present as extra-intestinal symptoms (symptoms that occur in areas other than the intestines).

A fine line can be drawn between the symptoms caused by CD itself and by the complications of the disease. The state of being unable to absorb nutrients through the small intestine because of the inflammatory process, resulting in damage *is* CD. In addition, however, it has been proven that, in CD, the small intestine becomes permeable (leaky gut) and gluten is able to pass through its walls, thus causing the complications that lead to other systemic conditions. We'll examine the known complications of CD in the sections of this chapter.

Known Complications of CD Inflammation

As CD progresses, it causes inflammation of the small intestine. The tissue of the small intestine weakens, becomes reddened, and the texture actually changes. This permits fluid and gluten to pass through the small-intestinal wall into the abdominal cavity and be absorbed by the circulation of the blood. This is known as a *permeable gut or leaky gut* condition and it leads to problems. The body only functions in a healthy manner as long as everything stays where it belongs.

Anemia

Anemia in people with CD is the result of the small intestine's inability to absorb iron. When the body does not absorb iron, not enough blood cells are created to carry oxygen. This causes the individual to experience extreme fatigue. Every part of the body suffers when it does not receive enough oxygen. The latest research indicates that CD patients with anemia have more severe disease than those who present symptoms with diarrhea.

Calcium Malabsorption

When the body cannot absorb calcium, the bones become porous and prone to osteopenia and then osteoporosis. A person with osteoporosis may suffer from multiple broken bones. Without calcium, the texture and density of the bones actually changes. If permitted to progress, the slightest impact or even an abrupt motion, can cause damage to the bones, or fractures. Also, this same mechanism is considered to be the cause of dental enamel deficiencies. In children, calcium malabsorption and dental enamel defects may be accompanied by other diseases. Rickets, caused by deficiencies of calcium and vitamin D, may be one of them. A study done in Saudi Arabia found that of 26 children with rickets (vitamin D and calcium deficiency), 10 were found to have CD. The authors of the study recommend that children with rickets be tested for CD.

Cancer

One of the most immediate concerns of all persons with CD is their increased chances of acquiring one of three different types of cancer: non-Hodgkin's lymphoma, esophageal cancer, and adenocarcinoma of the small intestine. These cancers may be caused by the constant irritation and chronic inflammation of the small intestine's mucosa or lining. When the proteins in gluten advance through the small intestine, the inflammatory process causes the T-cells to respond by multiplying. This increases the risk of lymphoma and the other cancers mentioned above. The only way to decrease this process is to eat a gluten-free diet (GFD) to allow the intestine to heal.

When a CD patient is diagnosed and adheres to a GFD, the risk of developing adenocarcinoma and esophageal cancer drastically decreases. The risk of non-Hodgkins lymphoma does not decrease, according to some of the research. (Some things in life we cannot control, and since research shows that mental attitudes do affect our health, this is the time for you to live life to the maximum in a GF state.)

Depression

The newest literature shows that depression is common among people with CD and that a GFD sometimes helps depression. Some people may need medication to balance the brain's chemistry, while others may need counseling. The important issue is to take control of one's destiny. A person with CD must be aggressive concerning improving all aspects of his/her life, including physical, psychological, and spiritual well-being. Even for mild depression, it is important to try to balance your life to allow you to encourage yourself, and realize the things that you cannot change. If you feel your depression cannot be controlled, do not hesitate to talk to your doctor or go to your local mental health center.

Dermatitis Herpetiformis

Twenty-five percent of CD patients develop a skin condition called dermatitis herpetiformis in which the skin erupts in a rash of small bubbles and hive like lesions. This condition can be biopsied and can help to diagnose CD. The skin eruptions are extremely itchy and are a manifestation of the damage that is happening in the small intestine. These symptoms improve on a GFD. Dermatitis herpetiformis is a *form of CD*, and actually not a complication. (For more, see Chapter 3.)

Infertility and Pregnancy

There has been more research in the last few years on infertility and CD, than any other subject related to the disease. When a woman is having reproductive problems, such as difficulty conceiving a child, carrying a pregnancy to term, or experiencing menopausal upheavals, she should ask her doctor to evaluate her for CD. When the body is not in sync because of CD, nothing works right.

Women with undiagnosed CD have a high rate of miscarriage. If a pregnancy is carried to term, an infant can be born with neural tubal defects caused by the lack of absorption of folic acid. Many women have gone on a GFD and delivered normal healthy babies. It is suggested that a CD mother breast-feed as long as possible because it has been recognized that breastfeeding delays the appearance of CD.

The most recent research indicates that about 10% of unexplained fertility cases are due to CD. Another study showed that 4.5% of those with reproductive dysfunction and CD that proceed with a GFD will then have a normal pregnancy. Remember, this applies to both male and females regarding infertility problems. Either party can have CD and have unexplained infertility.

Lactose Intolerance

It is not unusual in those newly diagnosed with CD to have lactose intolerance. Symptoms include: severe bloating, gas, and abdominal pain. Often, these symptoms resolve on a GFD. Refer to Chapter 4.

Menopause

The undiagnosed CD woman has a heavy burden to carry during menopause. By not having a diagnosis, the woman is dealing with celiac symptoms as well as menopausal symptoms. The GFD can help to balance some of the body's mechanisms while hormone levels are changing.

Neurologic Symptoms

Recent research on CD and neurologic disorders suggests that between 10% and 51% of CD patients exhibit neurologic symptoms, as opposed to 19% of the general population without CD. The wide disparity between these two numbers may be accounted for by different methods in how the research was conducted and where the research was done; recognized symptoms of CD may differ, depending on where the diagnosis is made. Research on CD is only starting, and all research results give us more parts of the puzzle that will eventually fit together to make a big picture.

In one study, about 10% of people with CD were diagnosed as having the following neurologic disorders:

* Ataxia (disturbance of walking balance)
* Attention deficit disorder
* Depression and/or anxiety (presents in about 20% of CD patients)
* Neuropathy (the loss of nerve function)
* Seizure disorders

Other neurologic researchers claim that the following symptoms are found in 51% of all CD patients, compared with 19% in the non-CD population:

* Attention deficit hyperactivity disorder (ADHD)
* Cerebellar ataxia (disturbance of walking balance)
* Developmental delays (children slow in speech and coordination)
* Headaches
* Learning disorders

It is important to note that these neurologic symptoms should never be brushed off simply as part of CD. Each symptom must be evaluated by an appropriate specialist. A neurologist should evaluate seizures and ataxia, while a psychiatrist should evaluate depression, anxiety, and attention deficit disorders. Neuropathy is a common symptom of diabetes and should be addressed by your physician.

Other Suspected Complications of CD

Other known conditions that may be complications of CD are still in the research stage. These could be considered suspected complications.

Liver Disorders

Several liver disorders have been identified with CD, such as:

* Increased liver enzyme levels
* Nonspecific hepatitis and autoimmune chronic hepatitis
* Nonalcoholic fatty liver disease
* Cholestatic liver disease

Cholestatic liver disease is the most common liver disorder among CD patients. This disease occurs when the bile duct from the gall bladder to the liver is suppressed, and the bile does not flow. In the majority of patients with increased liver enzyme levels, levels will normalize on a GFD. In addition, CD may be associated with rare hepatic complications, such as hepatic T-cell lymphoma. Because many celiac patients do not have overt gastrointestinal symptoms, a high index of suspicion is required to test for the CD and prevent serious complications.

Other Observed Conditions

Addison's Disease

Addison's disease is a rare disease involving the adrenal gland. Symptoms may include weight loss, fatigue, lack of appetite, anemia, darkening of the skin, sun sensitivity, low blood sugar, nausea, vomiting, diarrhea or constipation, and dehydration. The prevalence of CD in persons with Addison's disease is significant.

Autism

A study was done by Columbia University that indicates that those with autism spectrum disorder show an immune reaction to gluten. The conclusion was not specific enough to say that these children have CD or nonceliac gluten sensitivity, but they do show an immune reaction to the gluten. Parents who have maintained for years that their child had behavior changes by being gluten and casein free, will feel much relief. More research is needed.

Diabetes

Type 1 diabetes is present in up to 16% of children with CD. The nutritional needs of a child with both diabetes and CD can be a difficult challenge. A dietitian familiar with both conditions will be very valuable in assisting you to meet both of these dietary needs.

Microscopic Colitis

This is described as a patient with watery diarrhea but can also include cramping and is frequently associated with CD. There are two types of microscopic colitis: lymphocytic and collagenous.

Some of the research has indicated that nonsteroidal anti-inflammatory drugs such as aspirin, ibuprofen and naproxen have a correlation to this condition. One case study had a woman diagnosed with collagenous sprue whose GI symptoms improved on a GFD.

Other conditions frequently seen with CD include:

* Fibromyalgia (pain in the fibrous areas of muscles)
* Aphthous ulcers (sores in the soft mucous membrane of the mouth and tongue)
* Joint pain
* Down syndrome (It is estimated that 20% of all individuals with this condition have CD.)
* Dysrhythmia (an abnormal heart rate)

* Other autoimmune diseases such as:
  * Lupus erythematosus
  * Multiple sclerosis
  * Sjögren's syndrome
  * Pernicious anemia
  * Raynaud's phenomenon
  * Scleroderma
  * Thyroid diseases
  * Graves' disease
  * Hashimoto's disease

Nonresponsive Celiac Disease and Refractory Celiac Disease

CD patients who experience ongoing symptoms or persistent villous atrophy despite following a GFD for more than 12 months are classified as having nonresponsive celiac disease (NRCD). In many cases, NRCD is due to accidental or intentional gluten ingestion, which is resolved by identifying and eliminating the source of gluten exposure.

Refractory celiac disease (RCD) is a rare condition in which the body fails to respond to strict adherence to a GFD, and malnutrition and intestinal villous atrophy persists. Treatment requires additional, often costly immunotherapy treatments. RCD increases the risk of mortality and, according to a study done in France by Malamut and Cellier, type II RCD can transform into an invasive lymphoma.

CHAPTER 6

Tackling the Emotional Side of Celiac Disease

Happiness comes of the capacity to feel deeply, to enjoy simply, to think freely, to risk life, to be needed.
—Storm Jameson

Only another person with celiac disease (CD) can comprehend the emotional aspects of CD. Living year after year with a variety of unexplained ailments is extremely frustrating. Those who experience the depression, anxiety, ataxia, or mental fogginess that can come with the disease understand the significant impact it has on the individual and his or her family. It affects personal relationships, social situations, self-esteem, and confidence. The majority of people with CD have been told, "It's all in your head" or "You are a hypochondriac." Family members many times may have developed the habit of "tuning out" their CD family member when he or she has complaints.

Eric Cassell, author of *The Nature of Suffering*, describes suffering as: "A state of severe distress caused by events which threaten the integrity of a person." It could easily be said that "suffering" occurs in all CD patients *and* their families.

Many physicians are still not aware of the prevalence of CD. They are looking for other conditions such as irritable bowel syndrome, chronic fatigue syndrome, fibromyalgia, or Crohn's disease, just to mention a few. This only delays a clear diagnosis of CD and prolongs the suffering.

Common Emotional Reactions

Most newly diagnosed CD patients are subject to:

* Anxiety
* Insecurity
* Isolation
* Fear of the unknown
* Lack of information

Newly diagnosed CD patients need patience and understanding as they adjust to a new way of eating. This also applies to the parents of newly diagnosed children, who may feel helpless trying to find the information they need to have a healthy child. There need to be coping strategies and help with well-being for a child with CD.

Support Groups

Because doctors may not have the time to educate each individual with CD about the totally new way of life that the disorder demands, celiac support groups offer support among peers. There are many studies that show that those who participate in a support group are much more able to cope with their disease. One support group, the Gluten-Free Gang of Central Ohio, uses their group to discuss all new research, recipes, and restaurants in the area and offer support to new CD patients as they enter this new way of life. This group is led by a dietitian who specializes in CD.

Here is a transcript of a typical meeting of the Gluten-Free Gang:

"The doctors should address the extreme emotions we experience, but it is rare," Lisa told the group. "After I was diagnosed I was overwhelmed with feelings of guilt and deprivation. I felt guilty complaining because many people have a life-threatening illness, such as cancer or multiple sclerosis. I felt guilty because I spent more money on my gluten-free food. I felt deprived because I could not eat exactly what I wanted. Then my feelings jumped back to guilt because people in Third World countries are really deprived of food, not me. The deprived feeling continued for about a year. It was hard to watch everyone dig into my birthday cake, which I couldn't even taste. Then I felt guilty because I was behaving like a child. Restaurant eating was frustrating when I couldn't order what I really wanted. Then I was back to deprivation."

"My wife accused me of turning into a controlling husband because I wanted to become involved in meal planning and what restaurants we went to," Dean said.

"Things have gotten easier for me since I went to an open Alcoholics Anonymous meeting with my friend," Betty Jean said. "My friend explained that he could not drink alcohol because he would end up dead or in jail. He said I would kill myself if I did not eat gluten free. He showed a lot of empathy for my situation because he just had to stay away from alcohol and I had to watch every drop of food I put in my mouth."

"Do you suggest A.A. meetings?" a member of the group asked.

"No," Betty Jean said as she laughed, "however, I do think it is a good idea to write down the Serenity Prayer that is said at each A.A. meeting. Each of us can use it as we adapt to our new way of eating."

The Serenity Prayer

God grant me the serenity to accept the things I cannot change,
The courage to change the things I can,
And the wisdom to know the difference.

"I can use that prayer when I get exasperated repeatedly explaining the disease to friends and relatives," a new member said.

"Think of yourself as a teacher educating the general public," said Maryalice. "You are clearing the path for celiacs in the future."

"What do you do when you are invited to a friend's home for dinner?" the new member asked.

"You can still accept dinner invitations or go to a potluck, just bring your own food. Don't change your social life," Lisa emphasized.

Emotions common to CD patients as they struggle to adapt to a new way of eating include:

Relief at finally finding out what was wrong.

Grief over the loss of lifestyle and food.

Fear of eating something that will make them sick.

Frustration in finding the right medical help.

Difficulty in finding appropriate food.

Difficulty in reading and deciphering labels.

Difficulty in understanding and overcoming all aspects of depression.

Lucia, a member of the Gluten-Free Gang support group, offers this list of experiences common to all newly diagnosed CD patients:

Looking at a restaurant menu for the first time when trying to order a gluten-free (GF) meal, feeling apprehensive

(continued)

(*continued*)

because time is ticking away, silently shedding a few tears, and feeling as if the task is too big to handle.

Trying to decide on a snack or a packed lunch so not to be singled out as different.

Trying to convince family and friends that you cannot go off a gluten-free diet (GFD) "just this once" and "yes, it will hurt me."

Trying to explain ingredients that indicate gluten in labeling.

Taking two or three additional hours to shop for the family, and that before the trip to the health food store.

Making a daily decision regarding GF ingredients.

Individuals with CD must recognize that they have undertaken a new way of life. These complex feelings are the norm, not the exception, and fortunately, these feelings do not last forever. But because this disease is uncommon, you must continually explain it to family, friends, coworkers, teachers, doctors, servers at restaurants, grocers, and many others, almost on a daily basis. When you consider how many contacts are made every day, the challenges are evident.

"Don't think it is the end of the world," Mary, another group member said. "It could be worse. Years ago, people did not have support groups or health food stores that now carry numerous gluten-free products. For those celiacs who live in small communities, there are many Internet vendors who also sell gluten-free foods and also many online support groups and organizations to meet the needs of those with CD.

"We must remember to mentor newly diagnosed celiacs," Mary reminded the group. "I can remember coming to my first support group feeling alone, confused, and needing the help of others. I think one of the main shocks was when I realized how life would be different due to the diagnosis."

When Barb, the mother of a recently diagnosed child, walked into the meeting, the group asked her to share her story. When children are diagnosed with CD the parents need to make the largest adjustment.

"It is interesting to reflect back over the past two years since Natalie was diagnosed," said Barb. "So many emotions come flooding back. In hindsight, I wish we had pushed the celiac testing faster. We are in a minority because Natalie was diagnosed in less than seven weeks from the first major symptom, though she showed many of the classic symptoms from about nine months on.

"Dan and I had it pinpointed at about three weeks into testing by reading the *Merck Manual*, at our local library, after an upper gastrointestinal series of tests. The numerous tests scared us to death.

"My husband and I reacted very differently after the diagnosis. He was relieved and moved on. I, on the other hand, began to grieve for Natalie. I am getting better, but still have my days.

"I am already a compulsive person and, boy, did her diagnosis set that into overdrive! Nothing like coming home after the diagnosis and gutting your kitchen.

"One time, I remember we were nine months into our new lifestyle, and I was driving back from my first Celiac Conference at Children's Hospital. I just burst out into tears and had to pull over. I kept thinking, 'How am I going to make life somewhat "normal" for Natalie and our family? How am I ever going to learn all of this? It is so overwhelming.'

"I have since thrown out the word 'normal' from my vocabulary as much as possible, and my learning curve is beginning to bend a little.

"As parents, Dan and I have to protect Natalie while teaching her to protect herself from food. She has to learn how to live in a gluten world, and we struggle each day over how to teach her how to do it.

"After our son was born, a dear friend told me, 'Parenthood is a lifetime of joy and worry.' Boy, has that phrase taken on even more meaning now. When we have bad days, we always say, 'This could be a whole lot worse.' And we know that it could. We thank God for what we have.

"We are all healthier because of Natalie and we know it.

"The Gluten-Free Gang has been a blessing. Those of us with kids often struggle, since we are outnumbered by the adults. I have really focused on gathering up parents of children with celiac disease. Several are now coming back to the support group meetings.

"I also have tried to keep us all in contact via e-mail. With young families, it is hard to get to meetings, so we write each other as often as possible with questions, concerns, or just funny stories," Barb concluded.

Everyone at the meeting gave her a round of applause because, even though they might not have a child with CD, they were able to take courage, hope, and strength from her experience.

Support and Education

Living GF is a choice for health's sake. When the alternative makes you a high risk for several forms of cancer, plus other catastrophic symptoms, it is understandable that each day you must make a deliberate decision to maintain a GF life. This daily decision takes personal determination, family support, and a physician who is aware of how to treat CD.

The CD community offers an extended helping hand to new CD patients and to anyone who needs guidance in dealing with the disease. Information on physicians is available through the CD community, to provide patient education and resource materials so that appropriate referrals can be made. Great strides have been made in quicker diagnoses because more physicians are aware of the condition, but more education is still needed for physicians, other health care professionals, food service industry workers, and the community, as a recent study in Canada highlighted.

Many people with chronic diseases choose to go into a state of denial. This situation creates a condition in which the family must either "play act" to enable the denial or become confrontational and attempt to expose the denial. In this situation, an integrated health care team can identify the problem "up front."

Acknowledging and treating CD is important to avoid physical health-related complications but also emotional and behavior problems. In Italy, a study showed the necessity of diagnosing children younger and providing more psychosocial support because of the increased prevalence of emotional and behavioral problems in children with CD. In Germany, research noted that anxiety and depression were more common in women with CD than in the general population. Adherence to a GFD is essential to evaluate the psychosocial conditions. Continuing to eat gluten can make anxiety and depression worse. These studies demonstrate the importance of realizing that CD is a systemic disease requiring a full complement of care to provide the best quality of life for patients. The emotional impact that a CD diagnosis has on close relatives also needs to be addressed. Family members may struggle with the changes a GF lifestyle involves, even if they are not the one diagnosed.

A support group is an excellent source of information and encouragement. I highly recommend you join one. If there is not one in your community, start one. The Gluten Intolerance Group has many chapters across the United States. There may be one closer than you realize. It does not need to be a structured organization, just an opportunity for those with CD to share their concerns, thoughts, recipes, and favorite restaurants. Many groups even have activities planned for children, such as decorating GF cookies and lessons on reading labels.

Support is available. Find a local support group or connect with others with CD online. The Resources section will help you.

CHAPTER 7

Raising a Child with Celiac Disease

You give them your love, but not your thoughts,
For they have their own thoughts,
You may house their bodies but not their souls,
For their souls dwell in the house of tomorrow, which you
* cannot visit, not even in your dreams.*
You may strive to be like them but seek not to make them
* like you.*
For life goes not backward nor tarries with yesterday.
You are the bows from which your children as living arrows
* are sent forth.*

—Kahlil Gibran

Infants with celiac disease (CD) will usually show symptoms when grains (wheat, barley, or rye) are introduced into their diet. These symptoms will include diarrhea, foul-smelling stools, abdominal bloating, and probably abdominal pain. We all know when a baby has a "belly ache!" The appetite declines because of the symptoms. A noticeable change in the normal growth pattern will occur. It is not unusual for a child with CD to be in the lower percentile of height for his age. The general appearance of the child is what usually frightens the parents, because the child looks and acts sick.

A systematic review of available data suggested that the risk of developing CD may be decreased by breast-feeding at the time of gluten introduction. It is not clear whether this strategy prevents the disease or only delays the onset of symptoms. Gluten introduction should not be done earlier than at four months of age and not later than seven months of age since both early and late introduction of gluten have been shown to increase the risk of CD. However, several researchers have said that the longer an infant is breastfed, the less likely the child is to develop CD early in life.

Beth, a member of the Gluten-Free Gang of Central Ohio support group, kept a journal on her daughter and shared her memories:

"When Allison was six months old, she was experiencing bouts of vomiting and diarrhea. I kept pressing our doctor to find out what was wrong, and he kept saying that it was the flu or it was related to her recent ear infections.

"She also stopped growing, and she lost weight from six months to one year old. After six months of frustration, I finally insisted the doctor check her out. He scheduled a series of upper gastrointestinal tests. He claimed nothing was wrong and recommended no further testing.

"I called the Children's Hospital GI specialist's office and scheduled an appointment. We had to wait two months, since I was not referred as an emergency by another physician.

"Since she was still very sick, I kept a list of all medications, each doctor's appointment, and a food diary. When we finally saw the specialist, it took half an hour just to communicate the data I had accumulated. He examined her and said that he wanted to run a few tests to rule out cystic fibrosis, but he was fairly confident that she had celiac disease.

"My husband reacted rather strongly when we got to the car. He felt the doctor was a 'quack.' Even when the tests came back positive, my husband did not agree with the gluten-free diet. When we finally agreed on the gluten-free diet, our daughter began to thrive and started gaining weight.

"She looks and acts healthy again, and we are very pleased with Dr. Wallace V. Crandall, who is her pediatric gastroenterologist."

This story conveys some of the problems that parents experience as they strive to get help for their child. Parents feel helpless when they know their child is sick, and their level of frustration heightens when they are told nothing is wrong or they have to wait months for an appointment. If a pediatrician is aware of CD, the next referral should be to a gastroenterologist. The specialist should immediately order antibody tests and an endoscopy.

During the diagnostic period, the child may continue to lose weight and maintain a certain level of irritability. And the parents are, of course, under stress while caring for a sick child and frustrated because they cannot kiss the hurt away.

The parents' protectiveness often turns into grief when they realize the kind of changes they must lead their child through. Parental emotions run a wide gamut as they learn about the disease: They feel helpless as they search for food their child can eat; they feel guilt when they realize they have made a mistake and caused their child pain; at times, their self-confidence drops to zero. Every parent wants their child to enjoy a birthday cake or a snack after school with their friends. This is when intervention is desperately needed.

As a parent, you must recognize the importance of educating yourself, your child with CD, other siblings, family, and friends about a gluten-free diet (GFD), because your child's life depends on it. Parents or siblings cannot sneak "just a taste" of a donut or a muffin to the child with CD. Involve the entire family in the GFD. This will prevent your child with CD from feeling stigmatized. Make a list for family and friends of common products that are acceptable. Teach your family to read all labels, and celebrate family time and holidays without any emphasis on the GFD but on the healthy lifestyle that it offers.

Many conferences and support groups have programs for children with CD and their siblings and parents. For example, Nationwide Children's Hospital's Annual Celiac Conference organized in conjunction with the Gluten-Free Gang, a local support group, has age-appropriate classes and activities including how to read labels, identify gluten-free (GF) foods, and bake GF, among other offerings.

There are also camps for children with CD. These are wonderful places for a child to realize that there are many others with CD, and to enjoy and relax during mealtimes, knowing only a complete GF menu will be served. Activities are all geared toward helping the child adjust to the condition and become knowledgeable enough to live with it.

> Each child with CD should carry a short explanation of the disease and the importance of eating GF. For example:
> "I have celiac disease and it is very important that I not consume anything with wheat, barley, or rye, as the proteins in these grains make me very sick."

A positive attitude toward CD is extremely important because this is a lifelong diet. Support groups that have other parents of CD children can offer help, including:

* Education, including books and literature
* Recipe sharing
* Lists of stores to shop for GF
* Tips for snacks
* Emotional and social support
* Social media and research information

Knowing that others are going through the same thing takes away the feeling of isolation. Internet support groups are also essential, and can help you tackle the knowledge curve more quickly.

Children usually have the classic type of CD (symptoms of diarrhea, short stature, abdominal pain, dental lack of enamel), and parents can see similarities when they share experiences with other parents. A parent must immediately start building the child's self-esteem, even if they are still feeling overwhelmed and inadequate. Parents need to teach their children to adapt to various situations and to make every situation a teaching one so that the child's friends and family will understand the importance of following the GFD. This is when parents desperately need a support group.

Schools

Encourage your child to be articulate and confident about her GFD from an early age. When your child is in the first grade, she should be able to tell the class, "No, this is what I can eat, thank you anyway." Otherwise, she will always feel different and may be pressured into eating foods that will make him sick.

Both your child's teachers and classmates should understand your child's dietary needs. Make the teacher aware of what gluten is and what foods are allowed. Ask for a meeting to educate teachers, the school nurse, principal, and cafeteria staff (or other alternative, depending on the school). Take printed material describing CD and the necessity for your child to stay GF; having important information at their fingertips will help to prevent misunderstandings and mistakes. Be aware of special events at your child's school that may pose a threat to the diet. Offer to provide GF snacks so that the other children can experience what your child does.

If you encounter resistance or noncompliance from your child's school, or to ensure your child's needs are being met, you should be aware that Section 504 of the Rehabilitation Act of 1973, a federal civil rights statute, is designed to prohibit discrimination on the basis of a disability in an educational program or institution. This prohibition extends to any educational institution accepting federal funds. Students with a disability under this Act are afforded accommodations and modifications to their educational program to ensure equal access. CD is considered a disability under this law. Public schools and other institutions participating in federal programs, like the National School Lunch Program, must provide equal access to and participation in, such programs. Know your rights.

You may decide the best way to work with your child's school is to ask for a 504 evaluation with the aim of creating a 504 Plan to identify your child's needs, provide reasonable accommodations to help him or her succeed, and establish accountability for the school.

For more information on your child's rights at school and an FAQ on school lunches (visit www.americanceliac.org/for-families). This organization (American Celiac Disease Alliance) was responsible for effectively pushing the FDA to identify the term "gluten free" and label products that include wheat. It offers many resources on its website.

For a 504 Plan roadmap, instructions for teachers, and other helpful materials, go to www.celiaccentral.org, the website of National Celiac Awareness Foundation.

A positive environment will go a long way to allowing your child to be happy, healthy, and well adjusted. Teach him to realize that following a GFD will keep him well, prevent other diseases, and provide independence by being in control of his diet and disease.

School Lunch

In order to qualify for special dietary accommodations under the National School Lunch Program, a federal program bound by Section 504, a child will have to have his or her disability documented. Some states and school districts require a specific form while others require a detailed letter from your doctor including an explanation of how CD restricts your child's diet, foods to be omitted, and choice of foods to be substituted. Check with your school district. Though schools may choose to provide GF meals without such documentation, they are under no obligation to do so.

Snacks

When your child is invited to bring snacks to school or parties, many naturally GF options or homemade or store-bought GF alternatives (such as cookies and cupcakes) are now readily available.

Always have a GF snack handy in case one is not available. It is essential that your child feels responsible for what she eats. She must feel confident and self-assured in her decisions. Help her to realize that "eating gluten free" is a way of life.

Growing Up with CD: Danielle's Personal Story

"Hi, my name is Danielle Moore and I am 11 years old. I was diagnosed with type 1 diabetes at 16 months of age and celiac disease at 5 years of age. To be gluten free is so much harder than living with diabetes for now. It is a total lifestyle change. With diabetes I can push a button to give myself insulin, but there is no button to push to be 100% sure that foods are gluten free. My family has overcome the hardest part of being gluten free and that is the transformation of our lifestyle.

(continued)

**Growing Up with CD: Danielle's Personal
Story** (*continued*)

"My biggest challenge is school. I pack my lunch every day and I cannot participate with some of the school snacks that we have. My mom always makes sure I have a substitute snack in the class so I can eat with everyone else, but you are excluded from the group. Traveling has been OK. My mom researches ahead of time and always makes sure to pack food and snacks. Because I have to be nut and oat free also, we always are prepared.

"At first we were in awe of everything we had to look for and my mom broke down in the grocery store because of it. I thought it was too hard to comprehend. I quickly gained control of the situation and, just like diabetes, you have to beat the disease and not let it beat you.

"The regular grocery stores, six years ago, were not so gluten-free compatible, but because of living on a budget, mom was able to learn how to cook gluten free using what the stores offered and not visiting a specialty store very often. Nowadays, the regular grocery stores in Ohio are wonderful and have a huge variety of gluten-free items at a reasonable cost. I compiled a list of foods that we have eaten that we did not like so that we did not waste money on them again, another list with brands of gluten-free products that we like and don't like, quick recipes, and quick meals from the store that we can eat. I always make sure to have a snack available that is free of gluten, nuts, and oats.

"Being gluten free is easier than how some make it out to be. Mistakes can happen. It is very hard to be 100% sure that some foods are gluten free. If I eat gluten, I have learned not to get upset.

"Our kitchen is gluten free for the most part. My mom and dad only make one meal and it is gluten free for everyone. With work, school, and sports, it is too hard to make different meals. My mom will also make some meals and

(*continued*)

> **Growing Up with CD: Danielle's Personal Story** (*continued*)
>
> freeze them. We do adapt recipes to make them gluten free. My mom makes great cookies, pastas, meatloaf, and other foods that are gluten free. She also makes my birthday cake every year that everyone else eats because it is so good.
>
> "I love to eat out and we know a variety of restaurants that offer gluten-free items. My mom researched all of them, including their menus and talking to the managers to double check that they are gluten free. She now carries a list with her so we always know where we can go.
>
> "I do not stress about anything. I just go with the flow. I am 11 years old and this is my way of life. If you stress about it, the disease is beating you."

Danielle is such an inspiration and an example for many to follow, knowing that with education and family support the situation of living GF does get better with time.

Parents feel so strongly about protecting their children. The frustration level is high when a small baby or child is diagnosed with CD.

> **My Baby Has CD: Maribeth's Personal Story**
>
> "We were blessed with a three-week-old [adopted] baby girl who was the most beautiful baby in the world. We named her Lutricia. She was happy and healthy until about six months old. She would cry often after eating and by the time she was nine months she had diarrhea most of the time. The pediatrician thought she might be lactose intolerant. We took her off milk, but she continued with the diarrhea. After several months of this, we were referred to a gastroenterologist. She did a thorough history and did some lab tests, but she said that she wanted to do an endoscopy.

(*continued*)

My Baby Has CD: Maribeth's Personal Story (*continued*)

"The follow-up visit was planned for two weeks but the office called and said, 'We know you are coming in two weeks, but the lab work has come back and Lutricia has celiac disease. Take her off of bread and wheat products until you come for the next appointment.' When I asked about celiac disease they assured me that she would be fine and there was nothing to worry about. We did as they asked and found it rather difficult to restrict a sixteen-month-old from eating certain foods. We did notice that her stools were less frequent and she seemed happier within a few days.

"The doctor had a dietitian on her staff who took about an hour to explain what celiac disease is, what resources are available for gluten-free foods, about a support group that we could attend, the fact that there are genes that must be present to get it, and what kind of research is being done to treat the disease. The alarming thing that we realized is that the *only* treatment is a gluten-free diet.

"Lutrecia is now five years old. She is healthy, happy, and is in full control of what she is allowed to eat and what has gluten in it. The interesting thing is, she is adopted. I started having some gastrointestinal symptoms and I was diagnosed with celiac disease. That was the reason that we were unable to conceive. We are all eating gluten free and now I am pregnant with our second child.

Raise your child with confidence and encourage him to be informed about CD, empowered to take charge of his health, and willing to accept the challenges of life, not just the GFD. Joining a support group and networking with other parents will help you realize that you are not alone.

CHAPTER 8

The Gluten-Free Kitchen

Most of the shadows of this life are caused by standing in one's own shadow.

—Ralph Waldo Emerson

The transition to a gluten-free (GF) kitchen can be an exciting adventure, if change and choice are approached with the right mental attitudes. Each person decides from minute-to-minute, from hour-to-hour, and from day-to-day, exactly how to behave in a given situation. Each person makes the decision to either act or react. A reaction means we give the emotions permission to run the gamut. It can easily lead down a trail of anger, despair, agitation, and hopelessness. However, an individual can decide to be in control, to act and not react. Decide to pause and think about how it will feel to live a symptom-free life; picture the person you want to become, and then start acting like that person.

Make the decision to go down the happy road to a new GF life. Instead of becoming overwhelmed, let's together find a safe haven in a GF kitchen.

The kitchen is a safe haven for family and friends to talk, to share, and to eat. A person with celiac disease (CD) has the right to have a safe kitchen; however, it takes the cooperation of the entire household to help make the kitchen a safe haven for a person with CD.

Celebrate the new transition with dignity. Set a table with special GF snacks and light a candle. The light signifies the enlightenment brought into a person's life when CD is finally diagnosed. A light is needed to read and to gain knowledge. A light leads to understanding and consequently good health. It is fulfilling to enter the gluten-free diet (GFD) with ceremony and gusto.

The CD Safe Zone

Now, let's get to work. The right attitude is important as you prepare your kitchen. This is the beginning of living a symptom-free life.

If you live alone, no problem. Simply remove all items containing gluten from the kitchen and start from scratch. Thoroughly clean each shelf, including each crevice and corner, to help assure that you live a symptom-free life. This method is not realistic if other people live in the house with you, because you must consider their needs as well.

If you have a family or live with roommates, designate an exact area for the GF shelves and counter space. Several shelves and an area of the counter should be considered your "safe zone."

This special area is important because if a member of the family makes a wheat bread sandwich in the safe zone, and a few wheat particles from the bread contaminate food prepared for you in the same area, you could get sick. Make a sign to remind others that this is the "Celiac's Safe Zone."

Take the time to communicate with children. Make sure they understand the disease and what happens if food is contaminated with gluten. Children can help adults to obey the rules in a GF-safe kitchen.

All GF products, whether in jars, bottles, cellophane, plastic, paper, cardboard, or Styrofoam, should be marked with a colorful sticker or marker, without exception. Some people prefer to purchase matching storage containers. This method can be very expensive; however, a trip to the dollar store can drastically reduce the price. Jars with screw-top lids are airtight and allow GF flours to last longer.

No one should touch GF products without being overseen by you, the CD patient, or the person in charge of the kitchen. If a family member decides to borrow from the GF supply while making a gluten-containing meal, they could contaminate your products. Continue to explain, without hesitation, the importance of others following the kitchen rules so you can live without symptoms. It has been estimated that gluten the size of a grain of rice is adequate to begin the inflammatory process again in the intestinal tract.

Have a special place in the refrigerator to keep food and leftovers. Separate bottles of mayonnaise, relish, mustard, and all other condiments should be marked with a sticker or a marker. Squeeze bottles work for the entire family because knives or spoons are not placed inside the container and the top can be washed.

Porous pans, cutting boards, stones, or wooden bowls or wooden spoons should never be used in the GF area of the kitchen. Never use a food container if the interior surface cannot be scoured spotless.

Wash all containers thoroughly before using them to prepare a GFD meal. Stainless steel pans, skillets, bowls, and utensils can be used in both areas of the kitchen, if they are run through the dishwasher between uses. Stainless steel containers can be used to prepare GF food, and then rinsed out to prepare food for individuals on a regular diet. The whole household can use trays as food preparation surfaces, as long as the trays are washed in the dishwasher after each use. An excellent place to purchase stainless steel items for the kitchen is at a restaurant supply store.

The GF area should include its own pasta server and colander to use with GF pasta.

Since it is not feasible to wash a can opener in the dishwasher after each use, you should have a special can opener. Examine the cutting edge of any can opener and traces of food can usually be found. If you think it's clean, just use a toothbrush in some of the crevices—it is easy to see why you need your own can opener!

Keeping the workspace continuously clean is essential. Pouring cereal out of a box close to the CD work area or clean dishes can cause contamination. Family members should be asked to use the sink when pouring items from a package into a cup or bowl. This habit helps to keep any spillage contained in the sink. By simply running water, the mess can be cleaned up.

A single dad on an online forum for people with CD insisted that his three children use the sink when pouring cereal from the package to the bowl. They were also taught to open all boxes in the sink including crackers and cookies. He trained them to use a cutting board over the sink when mixing or cutting items for a recipe. He was very proud to share his story because this habit helped to keep the kitchen much cleaner than he thought possible.

Always place GF items to be warmed in the microwave on a plate, so that they never touch the oven shelf. You seldom see a microwave without a crumb. It is important to cover food with a paper towel, paper plate, wax paper, or plastic wrap to prevent food that is adhered to the walls of the microwave from contaminating the GF food.

A toaster oven has proven to be indispensable to many people with CD. The texture of GF bread makes it difficult to toast in a regular toaster; besides, family members commonly use a regular toaster for wheat toast. A toaster oven just for GF foods can be an extension of your safe zone and a good alternative to a microwave or conventional oven.

Shirley, a woman in her 50s, called me panic-stricken because she had been diagnosed with CD. Her life revolved around food: every Wednesday, her Bridge Club met at a different house for lunch and an afternoon of Bridge; every Sunday her family gathered at a different house each week for fellowship and to see who could come up with the most delicious and unique dishes. Every Monday was spent with the "Restaurant Rovers," a group of people who went to different restaurants to eat. She spoke about her concerns and confessed she had not visited with her friends or family while she converted her kitchen and was learning how to cook GF.

She had been quite verbal about her dislike of people complaining about their health. No one was aware she had any health concerns, and now she had to eat crow. She didn't want to explain CD to each individual member of her family, Bridge Club, and "Restaurant Rovers."

As we spoke, it was obvious she had a spacious home and enjoyed entertaining. I actually said very little as she talked through her concerns and came to a conclusion. She decided to invite everyone to her home for an evening of CD education. She asked me to speak. After I said yes, she asked me for an outline of my talk, because she wanted to hand out a brochure about CD.

Shirley's guests were impressed with the Italian meal she served that included bruschetta on rice crackers, breaded veal cutlets made with GF flour, and a crusty Italian GF bread. After dinner, Shirley's friends agreed to keep inviting her to all of their gatherings and not to be offended by her bringing her own food.

I must confess, it was an evening I will never forget.

Gluten Demystified

To learn how to cook GF, it is necessary to understand gluten and what it does. Gluten is the protein substance in wheat, barley, and rye that holds the dough together and makes the flour pliable and thick. It gives dough the ability to be kneaded and to hold air. GF flour does not have any gluten to give it pliability. It is necessary to adjust recipes by adding xanthan gum and extra eggs to recipes to add the elasticity that usually comes from gluten. The dough will be thicker, more sticky, and less pliable than a gluten-containing dough, but will taste just as good.

While there are some recipes in this book to help you get started on the new adventure of GF cooking and baking, a GF cookbook will be an invaluable resource for you. There are many excellent books available now, on everything from baking bread and sweet treats to making simple family meals. Some of my favorites, as well as several GF food blogs, are listed in the Resources section.

Essentials

Each GF kitchen should have on hand the following ingredients to make cooking and baking easier:

* **Xanthan gum, gelatin, and eggs** are used to hold dough together in all GF baking. Guar gum can be used but can cause diarrhea.
* **Rice flour** (brown and white), if used alone, will be slightly gritty and anything made from it will fall apart easily. (Brown rice flour must be refrigerated.) It works best if mixed with potato starch and tapioca starch.

* **Sweet rice flour**, also known as glutinous rice flour, is often called for in pastries or cookie recipes. It is lighter and sweeter than other rice flours.

* **Bean flours** are good if mixed with other types of flour. The most common are garfava (a mixture of garbanzo and fava beans), black bean, and mung bean flours. These are often mixed with sorghum flour, cornstarch, and tapioca starch. This flour is high in protein and fiber.

* **Soy flour** is a heavy flour with a strong flavor. It can be used in small amounts but not as the main flour ingredient.

* **Cornmeal and cornstarch** are ingredients often used in GF recipes. Cornstarch is commonly used for gravies and thickenings.

* **Clear gelatin** adds substance to GF recipes

* **Potato starch** is frequently used in recipes and flour mixes. Do not substitute *potato flour* which is very starchy, heavy flavored, and can be used in scalloped potatoes.

* **Rice bran, rice polish, arrowroot, nut flours, quinoa, buckwheat, chia, and amaranth** are also used in some GF baking recipes.

All the above ingredients can be found in health food stores and online. Asian specialty stores often carry rice flours. As GF foods become more popular, standard grocery stores stock more of these ingredients. All of these will be found in some of the commercially prepared GF foods.

Flour Mixes

When you cook and bake, you'll be using some ingredients you've probably never used before. There are many vendors that sell GF flours already mixed they all include some combination of GF flours including: Expandex (modified tapioca starch), potato starch, garbanzo bean flour, sorghum, fava bean flour, millet, and brown rice flour. Some add xanthan gum. However, it's easy to make your own flour blends.

Here are five of the most commonly used GF flour mixes that you can make yourself. These can be used for any GF recipe. By adding xanthan gum, these flours can also be used in baking to replace wheat flour cup for cup. Choose a mix based on your personal taste and availability of specialty flours.

Basic GF Flour Mix

6 cups white rice flour
2 cups potato starch
1 cup tapioca starch

Bean Flour Mix

2 cups garfava bean flour
1 cup sorghum flour
3 cups corn starch
2 cups tapioca flour
1 cup quinoa flour

Millet Flour Mix

6 cups millet flour
4 cups tapioca flour
2 cups cornstarch

Darry's GF Flour Mix

(from Darry Faust, *Gluten-Free Gang 2005 Conference Cookbook*)
Ingredients:
3 cups rice flour
1 cup com starch
3 cups tapioca flour
1/2 cup soy flour (optional)

Rita's GF Biscuit Mix

> 3 cups brown rice flour
> 1 cup tapioca flour
> 2/3 cup corn flour
> 2 teaspoons xanthan gum
> 1/2 cup potato starch
> 1 cup bean flour

The amount of xanthan gum you add to a recipe varies for different baked goods. Breads, which are high in gluten, require more, while cookies require less.

* For breads, use ¾ teaspoon per cup of flour
* For cakes, use ½ teaspoon per cup of flour
* For cookies, use ¼ to ½ teaspoon per cup of flour

There are many options when it comes to cooking and baking GF. Try these flour mix recipes or mix-n-match your own to find what works best for you. Even though these flours may be unfamiliar to you now, it is still possible to "make it work" and create delicious GF meals and baked goods.

Baking GF Breads

Bread is one of the most frequently missed items on a GFD. GF breads can be purchased from health food stores, some local grocery stores or through many Internet sites. Many varieties are available, both on the shelves and in the freezer. GF bread can be made at home either in a heavy-duty bread maker or with a heavy-duty mixer and then baked in the oven. (A light-duty mixer motor will burn out from the heavy mixing required.) When making bread, cut it when it is cool and place each slice in a plastic bag and freeze. When ready to use, remove from the freezer and either thaw naturally or toast. If you are using a bread maker, it should be programmable so that there is only one mix and one rise.

Buns

Making buns is an excellent way to satisfy a craving for bread. A bread recipe is great for sandwich buns. Buns can be made out of any commercial GF flour mix, homemade GF flour mix, or bean flour mix. Bean mixes are more nutritious and contain more fiber and protein, which is important because nutrition and fiber is sometimes lacking in some CD diets. Try to find a recipe that uses bean flours, sorghum, or a combination with cornstarch and/or tapioca starch. They will hold together better as a sandwich bun. Most GF breads, unless grilled, will not hold together well for a sandwich. Buns are a better option.

There are many creative ways to individualize buns, such as adding onion flakes, poppy seeds, sesame seeds, herbs, cinnamon, and raisins. Muffin top tins or baking rings (English muffin rings) can be used. The muffin top tins allow for browning on the top and bottom.

The same dough can also be used for bread sticks, cinnamon rolls, and pizza crust. The dough is sticky, because it does not have the gluten to make it pliable and stretchy.

All buns must be sliced as soon as they are baked and put into individual bags and frozen. This guarantees a fresh bun to satisfy the next craving for a sandwich. The recipe I've used for many years with great success in included in the Recipe section at the back of the book.

There are also commercial hamburger buns and hot dog buns available in the grocer's freezer.

Cakes

Many wonderful GF cake recipes are available. After a while, you will learn how to adapt regular recipes to

GF ones. Don't forget to add the xanthan gum (if it isn't already in your packaged GF flour mix). Cakes with nuts, raisins, carrots, and other dried fruit are more moist and stay together better. Cheesecake recipes are usually easy to make GF if you use GF graham crackers for the crust and many recipes are easy to adapt. Prepackaged GF cake mixes are also available. These are very good, especially when you are in a hurry.

Cookies

GF cookies can be purchased off the shelf at many grocery stores and health food stores, and from many websites. Many recipes are available for homemade GF cookies, too. Always use xanthan gum and never use a baking stone previously used with gluten dough. Except for stones, all pots, pans, and bakeware are considered GF after being thoroughly washed.

> Have a cookie exchange with your GF support group. Each participant brings a marked plastic bag with six cookies and the recipe for each member. Everyone goes home with many varieties to enjoy and recipes to try for themselves!

Puddings and Pie Fillings

Rice flour, potato starch, cornstarch, and tapioca can also be used for puddings and pie fillings.

Cooking GF

Though most people think of baked goods when they think about the adjustments to cooking and eating GF, you'll find that your flour mixes are useful for other, nonbaked recipes that call for wheat flour.

Gravies and Thickeners

Use rice flour, potato starch, corn starch, tapioca starch, or any prepared GF flour mix or a combination to make Hollandaise sauce, cheese sauce, or thickening for soups.

Breaded and Fried Dishes

GF flour mixes can be substituted cup for cup in recipes for breaded cutlets and batters for fried foods. The herbs and spices determine the taste more than the flour.

Eat for Your Health

Remember to keep a good attitude and decide to act—not react—to your new way of life. Make your kitchen a safe haven where you can enjoy your family and friends and know you will not get sick from contaminated food. Be careful not to make the GF kitchen a stressful experience. Words of encouragement to your family, including a thank you for their cooperation, go much further than complaining.

Enjoy a trip to the health food store and the Asian grocery story. Get a supply of prepared items. Some people will not want the full kitchen experience, but be sure to allocate a lot of time to reading labels. You might be surprised how much you enjoy cooking. It really is a satisfying experience to make a recipe with your own hands and then to receive immediate gratification by filling your stomach.

CHAPTER 9

Eating Out and Enjoying It

To be without some of the things you want is an indispensable part of happiness.

—Bertrand Russell

The gluten-free diet (GFD) is "doable" at home; however, it is nice to eat out, at least once in a while. The first time you go to a restaurant as a celiac disease (CD) patient, you might think you are prepared, but when actually confronted with the situation, you might find yourself overwhelmed.

Restaurant Dining

When a group of people with CD discussed their first adventure eating out after being diagnosed, they found some common denominators: an overwhelmed feeling when looking at the menu and not knowing how to explain your special needs headed the list. At one time it was helpful to use a card to explain what CD was and the need for a GFD. That is no longer necessary, as most restaurants are aware of the GFD though they may not be aware of CD or fully understand what gluten is, the danger to you if you consume gluten, or how to prevent cross-contamination. Restaurants no longer look with awe when you ask for "no bun" because of the low-carb diet craze and popularity of the GFD, but they may perceive the GFD as just a "fad diet" with no real consequences if gluten is consumed. However, the good news is that now most restaurants will try to accommodate your needs.

Keep in mind that, when dining out, there is a difference between a "cook" and a "chef." Restaurants that employ cooks hire them to prepare food according to the dictates of a corporate office, owner, or manager. A cook follows orders and is not always aware of all the ingredients in certain dishes. A chef, on the other hand, has been trained in the culinary arts and is usually aware of special-needs diets, such as those prepared for diabetic and CD patients. He or she is a professional who wants to create a meal according to the individual diner's needs and tastes. In fine dining restaurants, your chef may come to your table, discuss solutions, and make recommendations. Once you understand the difference between a cook and a chef, you can determine how to approach each dining-out situation. It takes time to feel comfortable, but soon you will develop your own way of handling the situation.

It takes confidence to speak out about what you need and what will happen if you do not get it. Don't get sick just because you are too shy to speak out or because you do not want to call attention to yourself. Be polite, but be assertive. Being diagnosed with CD is a great time for a shy person to visualize the person she wants to become and then start acting like that person.

Some national restaurants now offer gluten-free (GF) menus:

* Outback Steakhouse
* Bonefish Grill
* PF Chang's

(continued)

Some national restaurants now offer gluten-free (GF) menus: (*continued*)

* First Watch
* Wendy's
* McDonald's
* Don Pablo's
* Carrabba's Italian Grill
* Chick-Fil-A
* Subway
* Melting Pot
* Bob Evans
* Cecil Whittaker's Pizza
* Gatti's Pizza
* Sam and Louie's New York Pizzeria
* Fresh to Order, F2O
* Order Up
* Cameron Mitchell Restaurants
* Cheeseburger in Paradise
* Donato's Pizza
* Giordano's Pizza
* Mama Mimi's
* Buca Di Beppo
* The Melting Pot
* Pei Wei Asian Diner
* Ted's Montana Grill

And there are so many more too numerous to mention. Many local eateries may also provide GF menus.

Always ask for a GF menu. This will educate the restaurant on the need to provide one.

Your best bet is to find a locally owned restaurant where the servers are trained to cater to each customer's needs. If your server does not know the contents of menu item ingredients, ask to speak to the chef, briefly explain CD, and ask for help in making a selection. Once you know you are being protected from gluten, you can relax and enjoy your meal. This type of restaurant may cost more, but the extra money is worth the peace of mind.

It's not hard to understand why some restaurants refuse to commit to serving GF meals. As more research is done on CD and on the gluten content of foods, knowing for certain what foods are and are not GF presents a moving target. Research has proven that the proteins of grains used to produce vinegar do not survive the distillation process and therefore vinegar is now considered GF. Alcoholic beverages *without additives* are GF. Unless labeled GF, beer is not safe for those with CD as it contains barley hops. The ingredients in many prepared foods may change over time, and just because something is GF this year, doesn't mean it will continue to always be GF. One ingredient may change a formerly "safe" product into an unsafe choice. Don't abdicate your responsibility to ask questions and read labels to the restaurant.

> As of August 2014 food products may be labeled "gluten free" only if they contain less than (<) 20 ppm of gluten.

When reading a menu in a restaurant, look it over and decide what you want and how it will fit into the GFD.

* Rule out pasta, breads, breading, fried foods, croutons, flour tortillas, pita, or any other obvious item with gluten. (Unless they offer GF pasta and bread options.)
* For your entrée:
    * Do not choose baked meat, fish, or fowl without checking with the cook or chef first to make sure any seasonings (rubbed on the meat before baking or injected into the meat to enhance flavor) or tenderizers used are GF. Also ask if bread stuffing is baked with the meat, poultry, or fish.
    * Broiled beef, pork, fish, or chicken is always safe if the only seasoning used is butter, garlic, salt, and pepper.

* Side dishes:
    * A baked white or sweet potato is always a good, safe selection.
    * If in the mood for French fries, always check to make sure nothing else is cooked in the same oil. (This may also vary from restaurant to restaurant, so ask each time.) Oil used to prepare breaded onion rings, chicken, fish, or other breaded items will contaminate the oil with gluten and any food cooked in it.
* Salad:
    * Always specify "no croutons."
    * Vinegar and oil dressing is always safe, except for malt vinegar made from barley.
    * If another type of dressing is offered, always ask to see the container so you can read the ingredient label or, if the dressing is made "in house," ask for the ingredients. (Many a server has had to carry a two-gallon jar of salad dressing to the table for me to check the ingredients!) Most Italian and Ranch dressings are GF, but it is always wise to check.
* Dessert:
    * Crème brûlée is always an option
    * Most ice cream without additives is GF.

Most servers do not mind asking questions of the chef or bringing food products to the table so you can review the label because they do not want their customers to get sick. (Those who truly go out of their way deserve an extra tip). Remember, it is much easier on everyone if you identify your dietary needs to the server *before* the meal is served. If the steak comes served on a piece of bread, and you said nothing about your specific dietary needs, then it is your error, not the restaurant's.

The more you can help to educate the public about CD, the sooner safe (GF) meals will be served in more restaurants. That is a good reason to request a gluten-free

> The Gluten Intolerance Group started the following two programs to educate food service professionals and improve the dining-out experience for those with CD:
>
> * The Chef-to-Plate Gluten-**Free Restaurant Awareness Program** supports restaurants by offering training for staff and menu reviews.
> * The **Gluten-Free Food Service Management and Training Program (GFFS)** has become the premiere certification program for establishing best practices in gluten-free (and allergen-free) food services, with low- or no-cost solutions. This program helps food services of all types to set policies and procedures for controlling and providing safe gluten-free meals. This program includes onsite auditing to assure practices are being used on a daily basis.

menu at every restaurant, so that they know there are many who need it and to educate the staff.

No matter how long you are GF and no matter how hard you try to control what you eat, you are *always* at risk of eating gluten when dining out. It's important to be diligent. Even after 17 years of eating out on a GFD, I was recently reminded of this during a recent meal. I visited a local restaurant that had been highly recommended to me because their wonderful new chef understood the GFD because he ate GF, too.

My server was very attentive in taking my order to make sure it was GF. When my plate arrived from the kitchen, it had a roll on it and I *assumed* that it was GF. I also had coleslaw and French fries, which the kitchen had assured us were GF. I started my meal and had eaten about a third of the roll when my server came back to the table.

I said, "This is the most delicious GF roll that I have ever tasted! How did your chef make these?"

She looked shocked and replied, "May I have it, please?" I started to worry. "Do you mean that it's not GF?"

She hurried off to the kitchen and a few minutes later came back to my table to tearfully apologize. She felt terrible that she had not checked but I knew I would be feeling even worse in a few hours. I went home and immediately took some Metamucil but within six hours, I was experiencing abdominal pain and bloating. (There is no medically recommended treatment for an accidental gluten ingestion. By trial and error, I've found Metamucil helps the gluten pass through my system quickly while others I know use club soda.) The next morning, I was very bloated, my joints ached, and my mind felt foggy. Fortunately, this flare up lasted only 36 hours, but lesson learned: never assume, always ask, and always confirm.

> One of the advantages of being in a CD support group is hearing about places where it's safe to eat. Sharing these experiences, new recipes, and places to shop, makes the GF lifestyle a little easier.

Dining with Friends and Family

Friends and family can cause problems because they might not realize the dangers to you of not adhering to a GFD. You are sure to hear at least once, "Oh, that little bit won't hurt you, will it?"

At a recent International CD Symposium, Dr Alessio Fasano dramatically—and accurately—said "If you have CD, stay GF or you die." In a subsequent interview, Dr. Fasano further explained his comment. "People with untreated celiac disease have a higher mortality rate than people without celiac disease. If you have celiac disease and don't follow the gluten-free diet, you will develop complications that increase your risk of dying at a younger age."

Your response to friends and family should be, "Just as a diabetic cannot eat sugar, I cannot eat gluten because the consequences might be deadly."

It's a reply that might catch the attention of those who have failed to understand the importance of your GFD. If the individual still makes no effort to understand CD and acquiesce to your needs, then it is very important to not give in. Remain firm and continue to take care of yourself, even if it means not eating what is being served.

Always take food with you when leaving the house to eliminate the possibility of going hungry. Never hesitate to bring out your stash of GF food when others are eating things you can't eat. It is important for you to continue to enjoy all your usual activities. Just remember that the reason for any activity is to gather together for a common cause and not just to eat.

If you are attending a banquet requiring advanced reservations, simply respond on the RSVP that a GFD is required, and most large banquet facilities will comply. (On one such occasion, everyone else had to eat a pasta salad with dry stuffed chicken, while I was served a beautiful plate of roast beef and fruit. Being on a GFD sometimes has its perks!) In a small town or less-populated area, it may be necessary to take your own food. Remember, it is the occasion that you are participating in, not just the meal. Don't let CD interfere with your social life.

After becoming comfortable with a GFD, sit down and make a list of the most common brand-name foods that are GF. Copy this list and give it to your family and friends. Update the list yearly. They will appreciate your effort, knowing that they can take your needs into consideration when they are hosting a gathering. (They also will appreciate how many labels you need to read!)

A few organizations publish a shopping list that is updated annually. These organizations can be found in the Resources section.

Dining Out with a Child with Celiac Disease

When dining out with CD children, always take along their favorite finger foods so they will be sure to get something they like when they start eating out. Although most children's menus include many gluten-filled items, most restaurants will cooperate with you so that the child can eat safely gluten free. Always encourage your child to try new foods; this helps them acquire tastes for a larger variety of foods. (For more tips on diets for CD children, see Chapter 7.)

When Traveling

When traveling, plan ahead for meals, taking into consideration how long the trip is and what will be available at the destination. Purchase GF bread, crackers, cereal, snacks, and fruit. Pack a cooler so that an alternative is always available to fall back on.

CHAPTER 10

Managing Celiac Disease

It is not what he has, nor even what he does, which directly expresses the worth of a man, but what he is.
—Henri Frederic Amiel

The management of celiac disease (CD) is a gluten-free diet (GFD) for life; however, there is more to managing the disease. Be sure your management plan includes each of these six key elements:

C onsultation with a skilled dietitian
E ducation about the disease
L ifelong adherence to a GFD
I dentification and treatment of nutritional deficiencies
A ccess to an advocacy group
C ontinuous long-term follow-up by a multidisciplinary team.

Stay informed about the latest research on CD, changes in GF labeling laws, and other matters that may directly affect your health. Maintaining regular visits with your physician and dietitian to assess your symptoms and monitor for complications is essential. In children, this includes evaluating growth and development. Also monitor your emotional well-being; talk with a health care professional immediately if you are feeling anxious or depressed.

Day to Day

Managing the disease on a daily personal basis is the goal of all people with CD. Each day, you must make a conscious effort to stay gluten free (GF). Living a GF lifestyle involves:

* Reading all labels and knowing what you are eating
* Keeping a "safe zone" in your kitchen for GF preparation
* Determining that your physician is aware of the complications of CD
* Creating an emergency program so you have GF foods in a crisis situation
* Continually informing family and friends of changes in the GFD, so that they are comfortable preparing foods for you
* For parents of CD children, communicating with school teachers and playmates and their families to make food choices easier for your child
* Knowing the grocery and specialty stores in your area that stock GF products

---

At a recent CD support group meeting, Carolyn stated that she felt that, "Celiac disease is an ongoing challenge because of all of the variables and constant changes in items containing gluten." She said that even the manufacturers do not always know the source of starches used in processing. She also added that, "Many restaurants do not want to commit to what is gluten free."

At the same meeting, Laura said that she found it difficult to convince her family that it was a lifelong diet. Bob said, "My fear is that my daughter will get it." Ramona added, "I keep forgetting to tell my doctor to write on my prescriptions 'gluten-free.'" She said that she suspected she was getting gluten in her diet and later found that it was in her daily vitamin pills. Read *every* label.

Special Circumstance: If You Are Going to the Hospital

If you are admitted to the hospital, take an information sheet with you about CD that is available from the Gluten Intolerance Group at www.gluten.net. Give one to the admitting nurse and to the nurse manager of the unit to which you are assigned. Ask them to put it on the front of your chart. Also, ask to speak to the dietitian assigned to your unit. The GFD is much more prevalent today, but there are still many who are unaware of the necessity for those with CD to eat GF. Providing health care professionals with the pertinent information about your case will make it easier for everyone.

At the Hospital: Marge's Personal Story

Marge was admitted to the hospital with a fractured pelvis and a urinary tract infection. She is 82 years old and has been the caregiver for her blind husband, Bob. He is 91 and very alert and active. He has helped her with her GFD and they had converted their entire kitchen to GF.

When she arrived at the hospital, Marge was not able to explain about her diet as she was very ill. Bob was very proactive in explaining to everyone from the emergency department, admitting nurse, nurses on the unit that Marge was assigned, and the nurse manager of the unit. They were all very understanding, and some even had questions to ask Bob about the GFD and CD.

When Marge was able to eat, she went over the menu with the dietitian to make sure that what she was able to eat was GF. Because Marge was going to be disabled for a few months, the plan was to send her to a nursing facility for extended care. The social worker who arranged this made sure the facility was aware of her CD and included arrangements for her GFD to continue. Marge and Bob's daughter made arrangements for Bob to stay with Marge while

(continued)

At the Hospital: Marge's Personal Story (*continued*)

she recuperated. Each day that Bob visited Marge, he checked to make sure that she was getting what she needed. Their life together was making sure that she did not have to suffer the symptoms of CD by eating GF *all of the time.*

Educating the Public

It is true that the individual with CD must be responsible for his or her health and diet. But it's empowering to learn more about your condition and be able to educate others regarding a disease that they may not have heard of before.

Research into CD has increased by more than 200% over the last 10 years, and for that we can all be thankful. At this stage, education is the essential element. As newly diagnosed CD patients, their physicians, and other health care professionals are provided with up-to-date information, a more united effort toward managing the disease can be undertaken.

Future Progress in CD Awareness

As CD patients, we can all help increase public awareness of the disease by enlisting the involvement of restaurants and food manufacturer's to produce and market more GF items. In the past few years, we've made a few impressive advancements, but there is still progress to be made. Speaking with one voice, through a single representative organization would help:

* Establish the definition of gluten which is harmful to those with CD. The FDA has established that food products should not have more than 20 parts per million (ppm).

* Collaborate with the Academy of Nutrition and Dietetics to design and adopt a universal GFD (This is being done)
* Continue to improve labeling laws, particularly as they apply to medications. The American Celiac Disease Alliance and their CD Task Force have successfully lobbied for several new important labeling laws, but there is more that can be done.
* Encourage the American Celiac Disease Alliance to lobby for insurance companies to reimburse for nutrition counseling.

To accomplish these goals, all persons with CD in the United States must be united into a community that works for the common good. I encourage you to be a part of that community.

CD Abroad

European Union

According to the *Official Journal of the European Union*, these are the rules in Europe for GF standards.

1. Foodstuffs for people intolerant to gluten, consisting of or containing one or more ingredients made from wheat, rye, barley, oats or their crossbred varieties which have been especially processed to reduce gluten, shall not contain a level of gluten exceeding 100 mg/kg in the food as sold to the final consumer. (Note, gastroenterologists in the United States believe that 50 mg/kg is the maximum that those with CD should ingest.)
2. The labeling, advertising and presentation of the products referred to in paragraph one shall bear the term "very low gluten." They may bear the term "gluten-free" if the gluten content does not exceed 20 mg/kg in the food as sold to the final consumer.

(*continued*)

CD Abroad (*continued*)

3. Oats contained in foodstuffs for people intolerant to gluten must have been specially produced, prepared and/or processed in a way to avoid contamination by wheat, rye, barley, or their crossbred varieties and the gluten content of such oats must not exceed 20 mg/kg.
4. Foodstuffs for people intolerant to gluten, consisting of or containing one or more ingredients which substitute wheat, rye, barley, oats or their crossbred varieties shall not contain a level of gluten exceeding 20 mg/kg in the food as sold to the final consumer. The labeling, presentation, and advertising of those products shall bear the term "gluten-free."

Australia

They are the most strict regarding gluten in foods. They allow *no* gluten in foods that are labeled GF. They have a "low gluten" category of 100 ppm, but those are not considered GF.

Great Britain

Those with CD receive a prescription for their GF foods.

Italy

All children are tested by age 6 for CD. After the age of 10 they receive 140 Euros monthly for GF food and extra vacation for shopping for GF food.

Ireland

GF foods are tax-deductible for the costs that exceed the cost of normal food.

CHAPTER 11

Pulling It All Together

If you have knowledge, let others light their candles at it.
                                                    —Thomas Fuller

Living the gluten-free life presents challenges. A challenge is not necessarily bad; it can be good. The first challenge is to get free of the symptoms of celiac disease by following a proper diet, but this is only the beginning. The next challenge is the healing process.

As the intestine heals, the body is finally able to start repairing itself. Before you are diagnosed with celiac disease, gluten is preventing your small intestine from absorbing the vitamins and nutrients your body needs to function. Each celiac patient knows how important it is for all parts of the body to work together.

Yet the healing process includes more than the body. Integrative medicine includes all the issues that affect your health: family, activities, diet, medications, stress management, and exercise. Even behavior-modification exercises can help you change actions or habits that are hindering your health.

To maximize your future health and happiness, it is important that you make an effort to bring your body, mind, and spirit into harmony. It is important to get into the driver's seat and to go past the disease as an obstacle. This is an easy statement to make, but let's see what it involves.

Healing the Body

When a celiac accidentally ingests gluten, it will usually cause symptoms such as bloating, gas, pain, or mental fogginess, which may last for two to three days. Some celiacs do not have symptoms but are aware that they have ingested gluten. The first course of action in either case should be to take a psyllium-based fiber laxative immediately, which will help clear the intestinal tract and add bulk to your stool which will move the gluten through your intestines. This is not a clinically based prescription but a suggestion from those with celiac that this has helped. Another suggestion has been to drink some club soda. Drinking club soda will also help to clear your intestinal tract.

Follow a Healthy Diet

Because of the permeability of the small intestine with this disease (also called "leaky gut"), food either moves too slowly (causing constipation) or too rapidly (causing diarrhea). Getting enough fiber on a regular basis will assist you in maintaining a healthy body. It will prevent constipation and help with diarrhea.

Gluten-free foods are usually high in fat and carbohydrates because foods that are processed to *reduce* fat or carbs are likely to have gluten in them (read the labels). Switching to gluten-free foods can result in weight gain, especially in the first few years. Simple statements can't be made about losing weight; however, stress is also a common denominator for both the underweight and overweight. Others suffer from the opposite problem: weight loss. Nutritional drinks high in calories and nutrition can be used between meals to help you gain weight. Ice cream is delicious mixed with some of these drinks and increases the calorie intake. Unfortunately, there are no easy solutions for losing or gaining weight. Both situations are stressful.

Terry, from the Gluten-Free Gang, states that weight gain or reduction has been an ongoing endeavor for her.

"I've been overweight most of my life, except when I was real sick with CD," Terry told the Gluten-Free Gang. "As most of us do, I packed on the pounds after going gluten-free. It took a long time for me to figure out what I was doing wrong, so I've made a list of what was happening and why. Maybe I can help someone else to not make the same mistakes."

Terry's list

(a) After I went on a gluten-free diet, I was feeling hunger pangs as early as 20 minutes after eating dinner. Not because I needed the calories, but because my body was playing catch-up with nutrients.

(b) Gluten-free products are usually higher in fat and overall calories. If you eat the same number of gluten-free cookies as regular cookies, you will take in a lot more calories. When wheat flour is not used, the ingredients used to recreate the texture of the original contain more calories and fat.

(c) A lot of the time, I was eating the whole box of gluten-free cookies because "I could." Once I found a good-tasting product, I would go overboard and eat too much. Yes, this was definitely emotional eating; however, it was still necessary to deal with this issue as part of the bigger picture.

(d) Not that I want to make specific recommendations, but Weight Watchers has been successful for me. It is a flexible plan that accommodates my needs, and it really emphasizes healthy eating. There is no magic bullet to losing excess weight. Whatever method a person decides to use, it is always calories in versus calories out, healthy food choices to help the body heal, and activity to help the process along.

(e) I eat much less gluten-free bread and baked products than I did previously. This decision was not made because I cut my carbohydrates (carbs)—I need a lot of carbs because I ride a bike. I need my diet to include 60% to 75% healthy carb calories on the days I ride long distances. I choose more complex and unprocessed carbs that are gluten free, such as breads, brown rice, pasta, quinoa, and buckwheat cereal. These items contain a good nutritional punch. Certainly, I eat cookies or cake on occasion, but I choose foods more often on the basis of quality over quantity.

(f) Fruit and vegetables are friends. One can have a lot of "friends" for not many calories.

Work With Your Doctor

When you are first diagnosed with celiac disease (CD), you'll be preoccupied with the new gluten-free diet (GFD). Watching calorie intake is the farthest thing from your one's mind; consequently, if you've spent your whole life working hard to gain weight, you may suddenly find yourself fighting to lose weight on the GFD. This problem is usually not expected; it creeps up insidiously.

It is important to follow up with your physician on a regular basis. You will know by the symptoms if your intestine is healing and if your body is absorbing enough nutrition. Your doctor will evaluate all of your current symptoms, along with previous problems such as anemia, overweight, underweight, irregular heartbeat, diarrhea, or constipation. Continuous diarrhea may indicate to your doctor that there is still gluten in your diet. Constipation forces the individual into a continuous awareness of fiber intake. On the other hand, if you have *dermatitis herpetiformis*, for example, you may have lesions months after diagnosis even if on a GFD. Many celiacs have no more symptoms. Therefore, the symptoms you had at diagnosis should be the ones your doctor reevaluates in the follow-up.

Your physician will also consider the effects that CD has on your body and make a plan to evaluate them. For example, if you have not had a bone scan for osteoporosis, that should be done every few years until it is known whether damage has been done to the bones. Blood calcium, magnesium, folate, iron, vitamin B_{12}, and vitamin D may be monitored for absorption as proof of healing.

You need a physician who makes you feel empowered, since health is a state of well-being. Have a list of questions ready when visiting your physician. Continue to go over each question until each is answered to your satisfaction. Communication is very important, and if your questions are not answered, consider going to another physician.

To ask your doctor **before a diagnosis** or if you suspect that you have CD:

Why am I so tired?
How can I stop my diarrhea? (or constipation)
What can I do for my abdominal pain?
I have had behavioral changes, what causes this and what can I do?
I am so anxious and have an insatiable appetite, how can I stop this?

To ask your doctor **after being diagnosed**:

Would you recommend a dietitian to help me?
Which relatives should be tested?
What effect will this have on my long term health?
What should I do if I accidently ingest gluten?
Will you order the necessary blood tests to make sure that I am in compliance with my diet? Will you do this every year?
Will you write on my prescriptions that all medicines should be gluten free?

(continued)

> To ask your doctor **after being diagnosed:** (*continued*)
>
> Do I need a bone scan?
> Can I go out to eat?
>
> To ask if your child is sick:
>
> Why is my child so short?
> My child cries after every meal and is losing
> weight, what can we do?
> My child has diarrhea many times a day and noth-
> ing seems to help.
> Why is her/his belly so large?

Keep a Diary

Whenever symptoms appear and you are not sure if they are celiac-related, start a two week food diary to determine what is causing the symptoms. Write down everything that you put in your mouth. It may be a food allergy, a vitamin or medication containing gluten, or an item you normally eat, previously gluten free, that may have new or changed ingredients.

Improve Your Lifestyle

In 1967, Frank Speizer began a Nurses' Health Study (at Harvard University) with about 80,000 nurses participating. It was comprehensive and very successful because many of the nurses participated for at least 40 years. It started with an emphasis on women's health, but produced such comprehensive and useful results that a second study and a third study are being done. The most important result of these studies was to reveal actual lifestyles that lower the risk of diseases. By controlling activities in our lives, eating or abstaining from certain foods, or realizing and compensating for our genetic risks, we can become healthier individuals.

Exercise is probably the most underestimated activity that benefits the whole body. The intestinal tract moves more easily, the muscles are toned, the cells are nourished, and the body can maintain a steady weight with daily exercise.

Exercising is taking care of the body. All exercises should start with stretching. When you start to age, your muscles will degenerate if they are not used. Aerobic exercises help keep your body functioning by raising your heart rate to at least 120 beats per minute. The most recent suggestions state that 20 to 30 minutes per day of aerobic exercise is necessary for a healthy body. That could include walking at two to three miles an hour or walking on a treadmill.

If you are sick, being depressed and feeling inadequate are not unusual for a period of time. When overcoming any type of illness the mind becomes sluggish. Taking care of the physical body can help our mental attitudes.

Healing the Mind

Realizing that the body is controlled by the mind is the first step to healing. The rigors of everyday life lead us to be so "busy" that we fail to take the time to just "be." Savoring life instead of just rushing through it results in a more balanced life.

Time each day must be allotted to pampering yourself. Soak in the tub or stand in the shower and permit the relaxing water to help relax your body. A shower chair can give many of the same benefits as a bath. Water removes germs, removes odors, and cleans the skin. Each day you can walk into the water dirty and walk out clean. Taking the time to prepare your body for the day is a privilege. Knowing you are clean from head to toe gives you a confidence not found any other way. A tap of powder in the shoes takes very little time. Keeping the fingernails and toenails cut, clean, and buffed helps to give the body that finished look.

Now is the time to start the diary. Don't just use your diary to record the things you eat. Make a daily note of exactly what you do to take care of your body inside and out. This notebook could include any physical symptoms you encounter and what you have to eat at each meal.

Have you ever noticed that helping and encouraging others gives you a sense of self-worth? Bernie Siegel in his book *Prescription for Living* states that encouragement is "the helium of life." Experiencing CD can be a challenge. We have the choice of making up our minds to:

1. Live gluten free
2. Read all of those labels
3. Find a recipe that fits something that we really crave or feel deprived of
4. Find personal courage to not limit our social activities because of CD
5. Encourage other celiacs and feel better about ourselves
6. Have an attitude of gratitude
7. Develop belief systems that will provide us with confidence and hope

Become self-motivated. Determine what motivates you, look at what you value, and ask what is your purpose here in this life. Being thus empowered permits you to be confident and in control.

Thoughts have a definite effect on our body. When the body receives a message of despair, it sends signals through the central and autonomic nervous systems to *beware* that something is wrong. This can make our pulse rate rise and create panic attacks, anxiety, shortness of breath, and other physical symptoms. So how our mind reacts to things really does affect our physical health.

Healing the Spirit (Soul)

We are really three-in-one individuals because we have a body, mind, and soul. It is impossible to separate them (Figure 11-1). It is much more effective if we allow them to work together.

Researchers have diligently studied the influence of the mind and spirit upon the body. Use the power of this connection to improve your immune system and health.

Dr. Bernie Siegel asks in his book *Prescription For Living*, "What lifts your spirits and allows you to overcome difficulties?" The answer is very simple: "encouragement." Set aside a quiet time each day to contemplate your goals and plan for the day. This is a good method for obtaining control over your mind. Keep a record of your mental attitudes and how you are working to improve them.

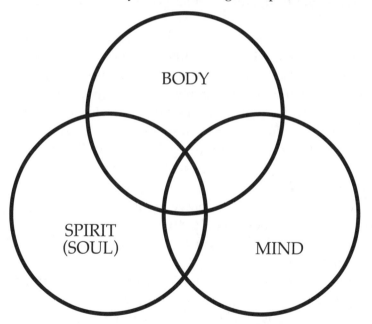

Figure 11-1. The intersection of body, mind, and soul (spirit).

Each person decides on a minute-to-minute basis exactly what they will think, what they will say, and what they will do. Each of us must take full responsibility for our own behavior. The mind is like a computer and the owner of the brain is the programmer. If you are not satisfied with your attitudes, moods, temper, or words, you can change them. Write down in the notebook exactly how you want to change. Visualize the person you want to become and then start acting like the person you are becoming. Set time aside each day to do this visualization, along with a meditation.

Dealing with family members can sometimes be exasperating; however, it is extremely important, for our own peace of mind, to realize we cannot change anyone except ourselves. If you want to change another person, try changing yourself instead—make an effort to act and not react. It works.

Everyone should have a certain amount of time set aside to enjoy or explore hobbies or interests such as arts, sports, reading, fishing, or whatever gives their lives fulfillment. Family members are not going to tell a spouse, parent, sibling, or child, "Why don't you take some time off just for yourself?" It is important to sit down and explain to your family that this is part of the healing process. Taking time for yourself is not selfish; it's just common sense. It helps you live a balanced life.

You can use meditation, prayer, yoga, or visual imaging to center your thoughts on something meaningful. These techniques will reduce your stress and increase your capacity for hope.

How do we deal with adversity? Remember, if a tree is not pruned, it will not produce fruit. We are spirits—souls. Our bodies can be crushed, but faith and love continue to be a part of us. As celiacs, we are physically changed (by wheat damaging our small intestine), but our spirits and minds are still intact. That is why we need to know who we are as a person—so that when anything happens to our physical body, *we* remain the same. Remember, too, that it takes time to absorb major life changes.

The most difficult person that I have to deal with is me. I have to learn to be honest and love myself as the creature that God created before I can set my other priorities in life. If you put faith first in your life, then personal satisfaction will permit you to put your family and other relationships in order after that. That will lead to a life of service and creativity, which is why we were created: to be of service to each other. This gives equilibrium to the body, mind, and spirit.

Dr. Dale Matthews, in *The Faith Factor*, states that we "heal the body by restoring our physical selves" and we "heal the mind by finding a lasting peace."

There have been several studies done to evaluate the value of prayer, yoga, and meditation on healing. In *Prescription For Living*, Dr. Bernie Siegel cites the example of Dr. Alijani, a devout Muslim who found support for his medical practice in his faith. He believes that faith plays a significant role in his patients' well-being. "On the basis of my experience, the mind of the individual plays a major role in the healing process. What stands out above all is his or her faith. If you have faith, you will be a well-balanced, resilient person, prepared to solve the problem."

Many people believe that prayer is a literal lifeline. Research has indicated that prayer is effective, whether the individual's own prayer or intercessory prayer by others. This is irrespective of one's belief system. There are many examples in Eastern religions of individuals being able to walk on hot coals or beds of nails with no pain because of their ability to control their minds. Healing is a state of mind that needs to be nourished and cultivated. Hope is the central path of healing.

We have a multifaceted body, and we are also multifaceted beings. The total person is not just the body, not just the mind, and not just the spirit (or soul). A total person is body, mind, and spirit. All three must be integrated and work in harmony for you to attain your full potential.

CHAPTER 12

Gluten in Medications

Steve Plogsted

Patients with celiac disease (CD) must be wary of gluten in pharmaceutical products. Gluten in pharmaceuticals is found in the pharmacologically inactive ingredients known as *excipients*. The purpose of the excipients is multi-functional. They provide bulk to the product, allow for the drug to be dissolved or disintegrate and absorbed at different rates in the body (as in extended-release formulations), decrease stomach upset, protect the product from moisture contamination, and simply make the final drug appearance more pleasing to the eye of the consumer. The shape and overall appearance of the final product also helps in identification.

The U.S. Food and Drug Administration (FDA) has the authority to approve all drug products produced for legal use in the United States. Each drug product must undergo rigorous testing before it can be approved for marketing to the consumer. The proprietary or "brand name" drugs need to meet standards for dissolution, absorption, blood levels, product stability, and several other factors. The manufacturing facilities where the drugs are produced must maintain specific standards in regard to quality control, cleanliness, and packaging. The equipment used to manufacture the drugs undergoes extensive cleaning and maintenance to assure that none of the products are contaminated by unwanted matter. Closed-containment equipment should be used whenever feasible and when not, appropriate precautions are employed to prevent contamination. Workers are gowned, gloved, and masked to avoid human contamination and to protect the workers from the medication. Many of the pieces of equipment are dedicated to one product, but if a piece of equipment is used for more than one product, it undergoes an additional level of cleaning and sterilization or sanitization. Computers are employed extensively to ensure constant quality throughout the process. The manufacturers must maintain detailed records of every step of the process and are subject to constant surveillance by various government agencies. There are also specific rules governing the handling of water and air in each facility to prevent any contamination from occurring.

The federal government also is involved in the content of the package insert that accompanies each drug product. The entire process can run into the hundreds of millions of dollars, which represents a sizeable investment for the drug manufacturers. Generic drug manufacturers must adhere to the same standards but do not have to invest in the research to the same extent as do proprietary manufacturers. The products do have to demonstrate that their action is the same as that of the previously approved proprietary product. This means that the active ingredient(s) must produce the same pharmacologic response, but the manufacturers are free to produce a final product that differs in shape, color, texture, and excipients. These products are rated by the FDA as equivalent depending on whether the generic conforms to all the federal standards for that drug product. Those that do not conform cannot be legally substituted by the pharmacist but can be dispensed upon the physician's authorization.

Excipients added during manufacturing may be from a wheat source including unspecified starch, pregelatinized starch, dusting powder, flour, and gluten. Dextri-maltose and caramel coloring, which may contain barley malt, may be a source of gluten. When trying to evaluate whether a pharmaceutical product contains gluten, the most obvious thing to do is look for the presence of starch. The word "starch" itself, unlike from the food industry, can come from any source. The most prevalent starches listed in the products include starch, corn starch, maize starch, pregelatinized starch, and sodium starch glycolate. Tapioca is used but it is not as common. Corn and maize starch are derived from corn whereas pregelatinized starch is primarily obtained from corn, although any starch can be pregelatinized and used in the product. There are several types of sodium starch glycolate. The most common one used in prescription products comes from potato. Sodium starch glycolate Type A and Type B are usually from potato although corn has been used occasionally. Type C can come from any starch source. Although sodium starch glycolate can be made from any starch, potato produces the best results when used as a disintegrating agent in a pharmaceutical product. Other starch derivatives such as dextrin and maltodextrin are usually derived from potato starch or corn starch in North America, and so should be acceptable for CD patients, but caution should be used until the gluten-free status can be confirmed. Several drug companies are using the wheat-derived maltodextrin when maltodextrin is used.

Pharmacists and physicians may often be called upon to determine whether a pharmaceutical product is gluten free. This can be a challenging task. In a survey performed in 2001, only 5 of 100 pharmaceutical companies had a policy ensuring gluten-free status for their medications, although many more stated that they believed their products to be gluten free. One of the problems faced by the pharmaceutical manufacturers is the uncertainty of the gluten-free status of the raw materials obtained from outside sources. Cross-contamination during manufacturing of the excipients can also occur but is very unlikely in the manufacturing of the actual drug product.

Over the past few years another excipient has been adding to the confusion and frustration when attempting to identify if an excipient is a source of gluten. Polyols, commonly known as sugar alcohols, are used frequently in liquids, but they are also common in tablet and capsule formulations. Sugar alcohols are not truly sugars or alcohols; rather they are carbohydrates that provide a source of calories. The sugar alcohols are naturally found in a number of fruits and vegetables and may be extracted from many sources including any starch, including wheat. During the manufacturing process they are completely refined leaving behind no gluten proteins similar to making table sugar. The mostly widely used sugar alcohols used in prescription drug manufacturing are mannitol and xylitol, however, others that can be used include sorbitol, maltitol, lactitol, and polydextrose. These products are used either as sweeteners in liquid drug products or as bulking agents in the solid dosage forms. The sugar alcohols are used in many diabetic products as well as in many health foods such as nutrition bars. Any person who consumes one of the sugar alcohols in significant quantities can experience gastrointestinal disturbances and diarrhea which may mimic symptoms celiac patients may suffer after being exposed to gluten. Regardless of the original source of the starch, they are purified to the extent that no gluten remains.

A reliable way of determining the gluten-free status of the medications that CD patients are taking is essential to their health. Several books and websites are available to assist in this process, but should be thought of as starting places. If possible, inquiries should be made directly to the pharmaceutical companies to ensure the gluten-free status of a particular product. Adding to the burden of the CD patient is the fact that pharmaceutical manufacturers may change the inactive ingredients of their products. This can happen without warning, so the gluten-free status of a product should be re-assessed on a regular basis. Any indication that a product is "new and improved," "new formulation," "new product appearance," or "new manufacturer" should be a sign that the gluten-free status of the product must be re-established.

One issue facing the consumer is that the pharmaceutical manufacturing companies may be providing false information as to the gluten status of their medications. One such incident involves a manufacturer of a well-known over-the-counter pain reliever who makes a product in a gel cap. The product is made using a polyol and a visit to their website will list their product as containing gluten. Although they don't test the product, they use the fact that the polyols could have or did come from wheat as a reason to label it as contaminated. Other drug companies have been known to label their product as contaminated with gluten when the source of the gluten is corn. To these companies, gluten is gluten and they don't bother to explain that to the consumer.

What does this means for the celiac patient? If you happen to contact a drug company for information and you are told that a drug contains gluten, you really need to push them to tell you which excipient in that drug product is considered the source of the gluten contamination. If it turns out to be one of the sugar alcohols you may wish to re-evaluate their response. While it is always up to the celiac patient to determine whether a product is safe for him or her the prevailing literature continues to suggest that these sugar alcohols are safe for use.

What kind of questions should you ask a drug manufacturer? First, you can ask them if their product contains any gluten. The most frequent response that you will receive goes something like this: "We don't knowingly use any gluten containing materials in the manufacturing of our product, however we can't guarantee that the drug is gluten free since we don't do final testing of the product." If you receive this answer, ask them if the product contains a starch. If there are no starch or starch derivatives, then the chance of gluten contamination is extremely small. If it contains a starch or starch derivative, ask them the source of the starch. If it is from corn, potato, or tapioca, then it is fairly certain that the product is safe, although trace amounts of wheat may be in any grain, even those that are guaranteed to be gluten free.

You have investigated all of your medicines and sources of gluten from food but you are still feeling your symptoms. What can be happening? There are studies that have shown individuals are reacting to maize which is used in certain drugs as a starch source and this may be what you are experiencing. Another source of the reaction may be the active ingredient in the drug. Although no drug actually contains the wheat protein, a common blood pressure medicine known as olmesartan has been identified as a cause of celiac-like intestinal symptoms. Researchers at the Mayo Clinic identified a number of patients who experienced a severe type of reaction that resolved once the drug was discontinued. Another source of contamination may come from the pharmacy that dispenses your medication. When a prescription for a tablet or capsule is counted out, the medication is placed on a counting tray from a bulk bottle and the specific number of units are counted and placed in the patient's prescription bottle. That counting tray may contain powder from previous orders. Although this would be an extremely rare source of contamination it is certainly a possibility which you should discuss with your pharmacist.

Very few medications are known to actually contain gluten and the chance of gluten contamination is relatively small, however, you should investigate all of your medications for its presence to ensure that you have done all you could do to eliminate contamination.

Table 12-1 is a short list of some of the common excipient ingredients used in the manufacturing of pharmaceutical products.

Table 12-1. Excipient ingredients in medications

Benzyl alcohol—Made synthetically from benzyl chloride, which is derived from toluene (a tar oil).

Cellulose (methylcellulose, hydroxymethylcellulose, micro-crystalline, powdered)—Obtained from fibrous plant material (woody pulp or chemical cotton).

Cetyl alcohol—Derived from a fat source (spermaceti, which is a waxy substance from the head of the sperm whale).

Croscarmellose sodium—An internally cross-linked sodium carboxymethylcellulose for use as a disintegrant in pharmaceutical formulations. It contains no sugar or starch.

Dextrans—Sugar molecules.

Dextrates—Mix of sugars resulting from the controlled enzymatic hydrolysis of starch.

Dextrins—Result from the hydrolysis of starch (primarily corn or potato) by heat or hydrochloric acid. They can also be obtained from wheat, rice, or tapioca.

Dextri-maltose—A sugar that may be obtained from barley malt.

Dextrose—A sugar that is obtained from corn starch.

Fructose—A sugar also known as levulose or fruit sugar.

Gelatin—Obtained from the skin, white connective tissue, and bones of animals (by boiling skin, tendons, ligaments, bones, etc. with water).

Glycerin—Historically, glycerin (also known as glycerol), was made through:

* *Saponification* (a type of chemical process) of fats and oils in the manufacturing of soaps.

(continued)

Table 12-1. Excipient ingredients in medications (*continued*)

---

* *Hydrolysis* of fats and oils through pressure and super-heated steam.
* *Fermentation* of beet sugar molasses in the presence of large amounts of sodium sulfite.

Today, it is made mostly from propylene (a petroleum product).

Glycerols—Obtained from fats and oils as byproducts in the manufacture of soaps and fatty acids (may also be listed as mono-glycerides or di-glycerides).

Glycols—Products of ethylene oxide gas.

Iron oxide (rust)—Used as a coloring agent.

Kaolin—A clay-like substance.

Lactinol—Lactose derivative.

Lactose—Lactose, or milk sugar, is used in the pharmaceutical industry as a filler or binder for the manufacture of coated pills and tablets.

Maltodextrin—A starch hydrolysate that is usually obtained from corn but can also be extracted from wheat, potatoes, or rice.

Mannitol—Derived from monosaccharides (glucose and mannose).

Polysorbates—Chemically altered sorbitol (a sugar).

Povidone (crospovidone)—Synthetic polymers.

Pregelatinized starch—A starch that has been chemically or mechanically processed. The starch can come from corn, wheat, potatoes, or tapioca.

Shellac—A natural wax product used in tablet or capsule coating.

Sodium lauryl sulfate—Derivative of the fatty acids of coconut oil.

Sodium starch glycolate—A starch that is usually obtained from potatoes but may come from any starch source.

Stearates (calcium, magnesium)—Derived from stearic acid (a fat; occurs as a glyceride in tallow and other animal fats and oils, as well as some vegetables; prepared synthetically by hydrogenation of cottonseed and other vegetable oils).

(*continued*)

Sucrose—Refined sugar also known as refined sugar, beet sugar, or cane sugar.

Titanium dioxide—Chemical used as a white pigment; not derived from any starch source.

Triacetin—Derivative of glycerin (acetylation of glycerol).

Silicon dioxide—Dispersing agent made from silicon.

CHAPTER 13

The Future for Celiac Disease

The man who cannot wander is but a pair of spectacles behind which there is no eye.

–Thomas Carlyle

The progress that has been made in the last 10 years in research of celiac disease (CD) and gluten intolerance and resources for people with CD has been remarkable. These advances empower people with CD to live better and share the knowledge with others.

The Future of Celiac Disease Research

Diagnosis

There is an evolving spectrum in CD and methods of diagnosing. In the future, algorithms will provide physicians a diagnostic tool to avoid the intestinal biopsy. If four out of five of the following criteria are met, then there would be a definite diagnosis:

* signs and symptoms of CD
* test positive for transglutaminase (tTG)
* either of the genes DQ2 and or DQ8

﹡ symptoms resolved on a gluten-free diet (GFD)

﹡ a biopsy showing mucosal changes

Researchers at The National Institute of Diabetes and Digestive and Kidney Diseases are studying additional options.

More clinical trials in the future will help us to determine more causative factors that distinguish CD and nonceliac gluten sensitivity. An increased focus in medical schools and an increased awareness in the public on these two distinct conditions are also important.

There are some new "point of care" tests for gluten sensitivity on the market with both professional and home versions, but these should really be read by a health care professional. Tests may be inconclusive, may have a false negative, and are not meant for a final diagnosis. Most gastroenterologists are skeptical of these tests for general use; however, they are here to stay and will probably be used for screening purposes.

Treatment

There is an abundance of research being done on a daily basis now for CD. Several drug treatments for CD are under evaluation. Larazotide acetate has shown some promising results in studies of diagnosed CD patients. Alba Therapeutics has announced positive results on the Phase IIb of larazotide acetate as a potential adjunct treatment for CD, in addition to a GFD. Note that the medication isn't intended to *replace* the GFD, but help prevent the autoimmune effects of continued gluten exposure as it works to close tight-gap junctions in the intestinal epithelium. While the study isn't big (342 individuals), the research was well-constructed (double-blind and placebo-controlled). Larazotide acetate is considered a "fast track" medication ready for Phase III study. It is very encouraging to think that someday soon, we may be able to take a medication that will assist the GFD in controlling the CD condition. However, the drug will not be available until more studies have been done and clinical trials completed.

Researchers are also studying a combination of enzymes—proteins that aid chemical reactions in the body—that detoxify gluten before it enters the small intestine. There are many enzymes and gluten-specific inhibitors available, but there is no research that, as of this writing, these are considered a safe alternative for individuals with CD. None of the enzymes available should replace the GFD. The literature shows that these are not effective at this time.

Additional therapeutic possibilities for the future are:

* Modified gluten grains that are tolerated by celiacs without creating villi damage.
* Pharmaceuticals that would inhibit the permeability of the small intestine.
* Transglutaminase inhibitors
* Deamination of peptides
* Degradation of the gluten peptide

Another avenue of research is vaccination. Nexvax2 is one potential option currently being tested.

Education

Scientists are also developing educational materials for standardized medical training to raise awareness among health care providers. The hope is that increased understanding and awareness will lead to earlier diagnosis and treatment of CD.

Clinical Trials

Participants in clinical trials can play a more active role in their own health care, gain access to new research treatments before they are widely available, and help others by contributing to medical research. For information about current studies, visit www.ClinicalTrials.gov.

I encourage you to participate in clinical trials. It is the most rapid way to find a treatment for our condition. There are currently 127 clinical trials in process.

The best way to predict the future is to create it!

FAQ

What is celiac disease (CD)?
CD is an autoimmune disease that occurs in genetically predisposed individuals and results in damage to the small intestine from the ingestion of the protein in the grains of wheat, barley, and rye.

What are the symptoms of CD?
Since the food is not being absorbed, the symptoms include anemia, abdominal pain, diarrhea and/or constipation and evidence of malnutrition.

What is dermatitis herpetiformis?
Dermatitis herpetiformis involves skin eruptions which are very itchy and usually on the extremities and also results in intestinal damage. It is considered to be CD.

How is CD diagnosed?
It is diagnosed by a full assessment, laboratory tests of a celiac profile, and, if these tests are positive, a biopsy of the small intestine by a gastroenterologist.

How is CD treated?
The only treatment, thus far, is following a strict gluten-free diet (GFD) for life.

What are the long-term effects of CD?
Following a gluten-free diet, the mortality is that of the normal population. If the diet is not followed, there is high risk for lymphoma, esophageal cancer, or cancer of the small intestine.

What is the difference between CD and non-celiac gluten intolerance (NCGI)?
In CD the intestine is damaged by the protein in the grains. In NCGI, symptoms occur but there is no permanent damage.

Do I need to repeat the biopsy once on a GFD?
Unless there are continued symptoms that interfere with your health, a diagnosis from the biopsy is usually sufficient. Most of the recent guidelines do not recommend a follow-up biopsy after following a GFD.

What is the definition of "gluten free" on food labels?
According to the most recent labeling laws in the United States, any product sold with a "gluten-free" label must contain less than 20 ppm of gluten, a level found not to cause damage to the intestine.

Is corn gluten free?
Corn is gluten free. It is only the protein in wheat, barley, and rye that is not.

Are oats gluten free?
Oats are gluten free; however, a study was done and 90% of the oats grown in the United States are contaminated in the growing or milling process. The only acceptable oats are those grown in a GF environment and milled separately.

Is coffee gluten free?
Coffee is gluten free (unless an additive has gluten in it).

Will I lose weight on a GFD?

The GFD is not recommended for weight loss. The literature shows that those with CD will gain weight after diagnosis regardless if they are underweight, overweight, or have type 1 diabetes.

How is lactose intolerance related to CD?

Lactose intolerance is frequently a side effect of CD. It usually resolves on a GFD.

Can my cosmetics, shampoo, or other skin care products cause symptoms of CD if they contain gluten?

Most physicians claim that the amount of gluten in lipstick is not enough to cause damage to those with CD. Dr. John J. Zone, a dermatologist who treats dermatitis herpetiformis, states that lipstick can cause a DH rash. There is no evidence that shampoo or other skin care products can cause symptoms in CD (unless it is ingested).

Recipes

The Gluten-Free Gang Celiac Support Group in Columbus, Ohio, participates along with Children's Hospital in an annual Celiac Conference. Each year, a group of recipes is collected from celiacs, which is then given to participants at the conference. When the Gluten-Free Gang was asked what should be included in this book, they all agreed that it should have recipes. After all, celiac disease (CD) is a diet-related disease and because there are restrictions, it is great to know some good things to prepare.

These recipes were submitted by our members as a courtesy to one another, and they include some of the group's favorite recipes. They are not meant to replace a cookbook, but offer ideas to the new celiac so that they may know that there are many options in preparing a meal. These recipes were reprinted with the permission of the Gluten-Free Gang website (www.glutenfreegang.org). Recipes from other sources will be identified.

*****

BASICS

GF Shake-n-Bake

(*from Jodi Carlson, 2001 Conference Cookbook*)

Ingredients
2 cups	Dry GF bread crumbs
¼ cup	Cornstarch
1 tbsp	Paprika

2 tsp	Salt
2 tsp	Sugar
2 tsp	Onion powder
¾ tsp	Oregano
¾ tsp	Garlic powder
¼ tsp	Cumin (optional)
¼ cup	Vegetable shortening

Directions
1. In food processor, whirl bread crumbs until fine.
2. Mix other dry ingredients and cut in shortening.
3. Store in covered container in cool, dry place.

*****

GF Fry Magic

(from Jodi Carlson, 2001 Conference Cookbook)

Ingredients

½ cup	Cornstarch
½ cup	Potato starch
¼ cup	Cornmeal
½ tsp	Baking soda
½ tsp	Xanthan gum
1 tsp	Salt and pepper

Directions
1. Toss all in plastic bag to mix.
2. Rinse meat to be fried and toss with coating mix.
3. Fry as usual.

*****

Thick Crust Pizza Dough

(from Darry Faust, 2005 Conference Cookbook)

Ingredients

1¼ cup	Rice flour (white or brown)
1 cup	Tapioca flour

¼ tsp	Xanthan gum
1 pkg	Unflavored gelatin
1 tsp	Baking powder
1 tbsp	Sugar
¾ cup	Cottage cheese
⅛ cup	Olive oil
½ cup	Buttermilk
1	Egg, blended with fork

Directions
1. Mix dry ingredients thoroughly.
2. Mix in wet ingredients.
3. This dough should be mixed and then formed into a ball with a rubber spatula.
4. Dust the dough ball with rice flour. Roll out on rice-flour-dusted wax paper sheet.
5. Roll to about 1/2-in. thickness (or about 12 inches in diameter to fit a pizza pan).
6. The pizza can also be cooked on a cookie sheet. Flute the edges of the pizza-shaped dough.
7. Bake at 350°F for 30 minutes.
8. Spread sauce over the top of the prebaked pizza dough. Top with your favorite toppings.
9. Bake for an additional 10 to 15 minutes.

✳✳✳✳✳

BREAKFAST

Breakfast Brunch Casserole

(*from Carolyn Randall, 1999 Conference Cookbook*)

Ingredients
6 cups	GF bread cubes or crumbs
1½ cups	Cold milk
10	Large eggs
1 cup	Buttermilk
1 tsp	Dill weed

1 tsp	Mrs. Dash seasoning
4	Green onions, chopped
1½ cup	Extra sharp cheddar cheese, shredded
½ cup	Green or red sweet pepper, finely chopped
1 cup	Ham, chopped small
10 oz. pkg	Frozen chopped spinach or chopped broccoli, thawed and drained.

Directions

1. Preheat the oven to 350°F.
2. Place the bread cubes or crumbs in a large bowl and heat in the microwave, stirring occasionally until bread is warmed through. Immediately pour the milk over the bread, stir well, and allow to stand.
3. In another large bowl, beat eggs together well with a fork or whisk. Stir in the buttermilk, pepper, dill weed, Mrs. Dash seasoning, onion, green pepper, grated cheese, meat, and spinach or broccoli.
4. Stir the egg mixture into the bread and milk, stirring to thoroughly blend.
5. Pour this mixture into a 9 in. × 13 in. glass baking dish coated with cooking spray and bake for 1 hour or until knife comes out clean.

Tip: The casserole may be made up to a day in advance and stored in the refrigerator, covered, until ready to bake.

*****

Corn Pancakes

(from Sylvia Bower)

Ingredients

2 tbsp	GF flour
13 to 14 oz.	Cream-style corn

| 1 tbsp | Vegetable oil |
| 2 | Eggs |

Directions
1. Combine all ingredients in a bowl.
2. Cook as you would any pancake on the griddle.

Optional: To "hide" corn, process in a blender in step 1.

*****

Early Wake-Up Call

(from Pat Rudolph, 2005 Conference Cookbook)

Ingredients
6	Eggs, beaten
1 lb	Monterey or mozzarella cheese, shredded
1 lb	Cottage cheese
1 cup	Milk
1 cup	GF biscuit mix
¼ lb	Margarine, melted
1 tsp	Parsley flakes
1 tsp	Dried onions
1 sm. can	Chopped green chilies

Directions
1. Blend together all ingredients and pour into 9 in. ×
   13 in. glass casserole.
2. Bake at 350°F for 40 minutes or until toothpick comes
   out clean from the center.

Tip: You can use ½ to ¾ lb cheese if using calcium fortified Lactaid Skim Milk, because this milk thickens well.

*****

English Muffins

(from Darry Faust, 2005 Conference Cookbook)

Ingredients

1¼ cup	Rice flour
1 cup	Tapioca flour
¼ cup	Powdered milk
1 tsp	Xanthan gum
2 tsp	Baking powder
1 cup	Cottage cheese
¾ cup	Water
2 tbsp	Olive oil

Directions
1. Mix dry ingredients thoroughly.
2. Add wet ingredients and mix thoroughly.
3. Form a dough ball with the mixing spoon.
4. Dust with rice flour to make a cannonball shape that rolls around the bowl without sticking.
5. Roll out the dough on a rice flour–dusted length of wax paper.
6. Roll to ¾-in. thickness. Cut out biscuits, any size. A 4-in. biscuit cutter will make about six biscuits.
7. Use spatula to lift off as the biscuits are cut. Reroll the dough as needed to make the biscuits.
8. Place on cookie sheet. Parchment paper works very well.
9. Bake at 350°F for 30 minutes. No need to turn the biscuits over during baking.
10. Cool on a wire rack until thoroughly cool. Keep refrigerated.

Tip: These muffins taste great when toasted.

＊＊＊＊＊

Gluten-Free and Dairy-Free Pancakes

(*from Heidi Hower, 2005 Conference Cookbook*)

Ingredients

| 1¼ cup | Bob's Red Mill All-Purpose GF Baking Flour |

1 tbsp	Baking powder
1 tbsp	Sugar
½ tsp	Salt
1 tsp	Xanthan gum
1	Egg
1 cup	Milk or milk substitute
2 tbsp	Safflower oil

Directions
1. Mix all ingredients in a bowl just until blended.
2. Cook on hot griddle until golden brown on both sides.

*****

Sunday Morning Waffles or Pancakes

(*from Darry Faust, 2005 Conference Cookbook*)

Ingredients

1 cup	GF flour mix*
1 tsp	Baking powder
¾ tsp	Baking soda
1	Egg, blended
1 cup	Buttermilk
1 tbsp	Olive oil

Directions
1. Mix dry ingredients thoroughly.
2. Add wet ingredients to the dry ingredients and mix thoroughly with spoon and let stand for about five minutes.
3. Ladle onto griddle: Pancakes will rise normally. Flip and cook both sides. Medium to low heat on an electric skillet works well.
4. Waffles: Normal cycle in preheated waffle maker.

See Darry's GF Flour Mix on page 92

MAIN MEALS

Aunt Carol's Spinach Casserole

(from Jane Ehrenfeld, 2004 Conference Cookbook)

Ingredients

10 oz. pkg	Spinach
½ cup	Mayonnaise, scant*
1	Egg
¼ cup	Grated cheese (cheddar, parmesan, or other hard cheese)
1 tbsp	GF bread crumbs or cornflake crumbs (optional)

Directions

1. Cook and drain spinach according to directions on package. (In microwave or on stovetop, it does not need to be cooked beyond thawed enough to drain.)
2. Drain all excess liquid. (I use cheesecloth and squish by hand. The more you drain, the better the dish turns out.)
3. Mix spinach with approximately ½ cup mayo, egg, and cheese. Can be done in the same dish as baking. Just wipe edges before putting in oven.
4. Mix a little more cheese (approx. 1 tbsp) with bread crumbs. Sprinkle over top of casserole.
5. Bake at 350°F for at least 20 minutes.

Note: A great potluck dish, this recipe multiplies well. A deeper dish makes a moister product (more like a soufflé) and a shallower dish is a bit more like a crustless spinach pie. Serve hot or at room temperature. Leftovers reheat well.

*Reduced-fat mayo works fine, but not fat-free because the mayo is providing all the oil for the recipe.

*****

Chicken Enchiladas

(from Judy Wells)

To make the sauce

Ingredients

1 tbsp	Olive oil
1 small	Onion, peeled, diced fine
1 tsp	Chili powder, mild or hot
3 to 4	Garlic cloves, minced
1 28-oz. can	Crushed fire-roasted tomatoes
1 tsp	Sugar or agave nectar
1 splash	Balsamic or red wine vinegar
2 tsp	Dried cilantro

Directions
1. Heat olive oil in a medium saucepan over medium heat and gently sauté the onion and chili powder for five minutes.
2. Add garlic, tomatoes, sugar, vinegar, and cilantro; stir; and bring to a simmer. Cover and cook 15 to 20 minutes.

To make the enchiladas

Ingredients

2 to 3 cups	Chopped rotisserie chicken (read label and confirm that chicken is GF)
16 oz.	Container of sour cream (save ½ cup for topping)
1 small	Onion, chopped
1 pkg	Taco seasoning (make sure it is GF)
2 cups	Shredded cheddar cheese (save ½ cup for topping)
1 can	Green chilies
	Corn tortillas

Directions
1. Heat oven to 350°F.
2. Combine chicken, 1½ cup sour cream, taco seasoning, chilies, and 1½ cup cheddar cheese.
3. Spoon about ¼ cup chicken mixture down center of tortilla; roll up. Place, seam-side down, in 13 in. × 9 in. baking dish; top with Quickie Enchilada Sauce.
4. Bake 30 to 45 minutes. Sprinkle with remaining cheese; bake five minutes or until cheese is melted.
5. Top with lettuce, tomatoes, black olives, and remaining sour cream.

*****

Chicken Salad

(from Judy Wells)

Ingredients

2½ cups	Diced cooked chicken (such as leftover rotisserie chicken)
1 cup	Celery, finely chopped
1 cup	Seedless red grapes, halved
1 cup	Pecans, lightly chopped
1 small	Onion, grated
½ cup	Mayonnaise
	Salt and pepper to taste

Directions
1. Mix all ingredients and chill until ready to serve.

*****

Corn Tortilla Pizza

(from Mary Anderson, 2004 Conference Cookbook)

Ingredients

2	Corn tortillas
	Salsa
	Toppings, as desired

Directions
1. Put sauce between the tortillas to hold together.
2. Top with your favorite pizza toppings.
3. Bake 10 to 12 minutes.

Money-saving tip: Instead of ready-made pizza shells use corn tortillas. One package of 10 will yield 5 small pizzas.

*****

Crunchy Chicken Nuggets

(from Jan Bowne, 1999 Conference Cookbook)

Ingredients

2 whole	Boneless, skinless chicken breasts, cut into 1½- to 2-in. cubes
¼ cup	Rice flour
¼ tsp	Paprika
⅛ tsp	Pepper
1	Egg, beaten
2 tbsp	Milk
½ cup	GF bread crumbs, toasted

Directions
1. Combine flour, paprika, and pepper in large resealable plastic bag.
2. Add chicken cubes, close, and shake to coat evenly.
3. In a small bowl, combine egg and milk. Dip coated cubes into egg mixture.
4. In another resealable plastic bag, place bread crumbs and add cubes to coat.
5. Place on baking sheet, bake at 400°F for 10 to 20 minutes.

*****

Eggplant Parmesan

(from Sherry Weinstein, 2004 Conference Cookbook)
Makes about four main servings

Ingredients

1 large	Eggplant
1 large	Egg, or 2 egg whites
1 cup	Parmesan cheese
½ jar	Spaghetti sauce
1 cup	Shredded mozzarella cheese
¾ tsp	Dried basil
	Additional Parmesan cheese for topping

Directions

1. Cut eggplant lengthwise into ½-in. thick slices.
2. In pie plate, beat egg with 1 to 2 tbsp water until blended.
3. In another bowl, mix Parmesan cheese and basil. Dip eggplant slices in egg mixture, then coat with Parmesan mixture.
4. Arrange enough coated eggplant to fit in single layer on large cookie sheet.
5. Broil 10 to 12 minutes or until lightly browned on both sides, turning once.
6. Remove eggplant to plate. Repeat with remaining eggplant.
7. Adjust oven temperature to 400°F.
8. In 9 in. × 13 in. baking dish, spoon some of the sauce and top with half of broiled eggplant, slightly overlapping.
9. Layer half of remaining sauce and half of the Parmesan cheese. Repeat layering and sprinkle top with grated Parmesan cheese.
10. Recipe can easily be doubled using two medium-sized eggplants.

Note: This is a light version, since the eggplant is broiled instead of fried. The dish, which always wins raves, substitutes parmesan cheese for the traditionally used bread crumbs to coat the eggplant.

*****

GF Lasagna

(from Mary Anderson, 2005 Conference Cookbook)

Ingredients

1 lb	Ground beef, cooked and drained
1 jar	Your favorite GF spaghetti sauce or homemade sauce
6	GF lasagna noodles, cooked *al dente*
1	Egg, beaten
2 cups	Cottage cheese
½ cup	Grated parmesan cheese
8 oz.	Sliced mozzarella cheese
1 tbsp	Dried parsley flakes

Directions
1. Preheat oven to 350°F.
2. Combine egg, cottage cheese, ¼ cup parmesan cheese, and parsley flakes.
3. Combine ground beef and sauce.
4. Layer half of the cooked noodles in 13 in. × 9 in. baking dish.
5. Spread half the cottage cheese mixture over noodles, then half the sauce mixture.
6. Top with half the mozzarella cheese. Repeat layers.
7. Sprinkle remaining parmesan cheese on top.
8. Bake for 40 minutes.

*****

Impossible Chicken 'n Broccoli Pie

(from Sylvia Bower)
Makes 6 to 8 servings

Ingredients

10 oz.	Frozen chopped broccoli
3 cups	Shredded cheddar cheese
1½ cups	Cooked chicken, cut up

⅔ cup	Chopped onion
1⅓ cups	Milk
3	Eggs
¾ cup	GF biscuit mix
¾ tsp	Salt
¼ tsp	Pepper

Directions
1. Heat oven to 400°F.
2. Grease 10 in. × 11½ in. pie plate.
3. Rinse frozen broccoli under running water to thaw. Drain thoroughly.
4. Mix broccoli, 2 cups cheese, chicken, and onions in pie plate.
5. Beat milk, eggs, baking mix, salt, and pepper until smooth—15 seconds in blender or one minute with hand mixer.
6. Pour into pie plate.
7. Bake 25 to 35 minutes, until knife inserted in center comes out clean.
8. Top with remaining cheese.
9. Bake one to two minutes longer, until cheese is melted.
10. Cool five minutes.

*****

Jamaican Jerk Chicken

(from Bob Janosy, 2004 Conference Cookbook)

Ingredients

6	Scallions, green only, sliced thin
2 large	Shallots, finely minced
2 large	Cloves garlic, finely minced
1 tbsp	Fresh ginger, finely minced
1 tsp	Hot fresh chili pepper (Scotch bonnet or habanero), seeded, finely chopped
1 tbsp	Ground allspice
1 tsp	Fresh ground black pepper

¼ tsp	Cayenne pepper
1 tsp	Ground cinnamon
½ tsp	Ground nutmeg
1 tbsp	Fresh thyme or 1 tsp dried
1 tsp	Coarse salt
1 tbsp	Dark brown sugar
½ cup	Fresh orange juice
½ cup	Rice vinegar
¼ cup	Red wine vinegar
¼ cup	Soy sauce
¼ cup	Olive oil
2 whole	Chickens, quartered

Directions
1. In a small bowl, combine scallions, shallots, garlic, ginger, and chili.
2. In another bowl, combine spices, salt, and sugar. Mix thoroughly.
3. Whisk in orange juice, vinegars, and soy sauce.
4. Slowly drizzle in oil, whisking constantly.
5. Add reserved scallion mixture and stir. Let rest one hour.
6. Wash chicken and place in bowl.
7. Add sauce to chicken and rub in well (use gloves to protect hands from hot chilies).
8. Cover and refrigerate overnight.
9. Cook the chicken in a skillet with small amount of oil until tender.

*****

Polenta Lasagna

(from Denise Loehr, 2004 Conference Cookbook)

Ingredients
1 tube	Polenta
	Cooking spray
15 oz.	Ricotta cheese
½ tsp	Crushed red pepper

10 oz.	Frozen chopped spinach
2	Egg whites
1 jar	Marinara sauce
1 cup	Parmesan cheese, fresh preshredded

Directions
1. Preheat oven to 400°F.
2. Spray 11 in. × 7 in. baking sheet with cooking spray.
3. Cut polenta in ½-in. width and arrange on pan to form bottom layer.
4. Mix together ricotta cheese, red pepper, spinach, and egg. Spread over polenta.
5. Spoon marinara sauce on top evenly.
6. Cover with foil and bake for 30 minutes.
7. Uncover and sprinkle with cheese and bake for additional five minutes or until cheese melts.

*****

Spinach Pie (Quiche)

(from Puri Purta, 2005 Conference Cookbook)

Ingredients

10-oz. pkg	Frozen spinach
3	Eggs
12 oz.	Cottage cheese
3 tbsp	Buckwheat flour
2 tbsp	Butter, melted
1 cup	Cheddar cheese, grated

Directions
1. Preheat oven to 350°F.
2. Thaw spinach, squeeze out water, and chop.
3. Mix all the ingredients together.
4. Spray deep dish pie pan or square 9 in. × 9 in. pan with no-stick spray (such as Pam). Pour mixture.
5. Bake for 45 minutes to one hour until edges are brown.

*****

Spring Mix Salad

(from Judy Wells)

Ingredients

1 bag	Spring Mix prepared greens
1 cup	Walnuts
1 can	Mandarin oranges
1 cup	Dried apricots, chopped
	Shredded (leftover) rotisserie chicken

Directions

Assemble walnuts, oranges, apricots, and shredded chicken over the salad greens. Top with your favorite dressing.

*****

Sweet and Sour Pork

(from Becky Paloci, 1999 Conference Cookbook)

Ingredients

1½ lb	Pork, cut in cubes
2-lb can	Pineapple chunks
¼ cup	Brown sugar
2 tbsp	Cornstarch
¼ cup	Cider vinegar
2 to 3 tbsp	GF soy sauce
½ tsp	Salt
1	Green pepper, cut into strips
¼ cup	Onion, thinly sliced

Directions

1. Brown pork, add ½ cup water. Cover and simmer until tender, about one hour.
2. Drain pineapple and reserve juice.
3. Combine brown sugar, cornstarch, pineapple juice, vinegar, soy sauce, and salt.
4. Add to pork, cook, and stir until gravy thickens.

5. Add pineapple, green pepper, and onion.

6. Cook two to three minutes. Serve over rice.

Tip: This recipe was one my mother always made and it is wonderful! You also can use a pressure cooker for the pork or cook it in electric skillet or crock pot.

*****

SOUPS

Chinese Corn Soup

(from Karen Hutson, 2005 Conference Cookbook)

Ingredients

2	Whole chicken breasts, boned and skinned
1	Egg white
1 tbsp	Rice wine
1 tbsp	Cornstarch
1 qt	Chicken stock
8 oz. can	Creamed corn
1 tsp	Salt
1½ tsp	Pepper
1	Egg, beaten
2 tbsp	Cornstarch dissolved in 2 tbsp water

Directions

1. Dice chicken into bite-sized pieces or slice to thin slivers and combine with the egg white, rice wine, and cornstarch. Set aside.

2. Bring to a boil the chicken stock, creamed corn, salt, and pepper.

3. When stock reaches a boil, add chicken, stirring constantly to break up chicken. Cook one minute.

4. Add egg in a thin stream, stirring slowly in one direction. Stir in cornstarch/water mixture. Cook one to two minutes.

Tip: If chicken stock is already salted, reduce salt in step 2.

*****

Susan's Potato Soup

(from Mary Louise McNamara, 2004 Conference Cookbook)

Ingredients

4	Potatoes, peeled and chopped
¼ cup	Celery, chopped
¼ cup	Onion, chopped
1 tsp	Parsley flakes
1 cube	Chicken bouillon (optional)
½ tsp	Salt
1½ cup	Milk
½ lb	Velveeta, cubed
2 tbsp	GF flour (optional)
	Pepper to taste

Directions
1. In a large saucepan, bring to boil (with just enough water to cover) potatoes, celery, onion, parsley, bouillon cube, and seasonings.
2. Mix well, cover, and simmer until tender.
3. Mix milk and flour together and add to veggies.
4. Cook until thickened. Add cheese and stir until melted.
5. The cheese thickens the soup.

Note: Ham can be added!

*****

Tortilla Soup

(from Sandy Izsak, 2004 Conference Cookbook)

Ingredients

	6-in. corn tortillas
3 large	Tomatoes, chopped (3 cups)
4 medium	Carrots, sliced (2 cups)
1 large	Onion, chopped (1 cup)

1 cup	Water
14½ oz. can	Chicken broth
4½ oz. can	Chopped green chili peppers
2 tsp	Chili powder
⅛ tsp	Salt
15-oz. can	Pinto beans, rinsed and drained
⅓ cup	Snipped fresh cilantro
	Tabasco to taste (optional)

Directions
1. Cut tortillas into ½-in. strips and cut in half crosswise.
2. Place on ungreased baking sheet. Bake 350°F for 10 to 13 minutes.
3. Set aside.
4. Combine all ingredients except for pinto beans and cilantro.
5. Bring to a boil, reduce heat, and simmer covered for 20 minutes.
6. Add beans and cilantro. Heat through.
7. Ladle soup into bowls. Divide strips among bowls.
8. Serve immediately.

*****

SALADS

Bean Salad

(from Carol Kimball, 2002 Conference Cookbook)

Ingredients

1 can	Kidney beans
1 can	Wax beans
1 can	Green beans
1 medium	Onion, chopped
1	Green pepper, chopped
1 cup	Celery, chopped
1 cup	Vinegar

1 tbsp	Water
1/3 cup	Oil
1 cup	Sugar
1 tsp	Salt
1 tsp	Paprika

Directions
1. Make salad dressing by whisking together vinegar, water, oil, sugar, salt, and paprika.
2. Coat beans, onion, pepper, and celery with the dressing and serve chilled.

*****

Broccoli Salad

(from Mary Anderson, 2005 Conference Cookbook)

Ingredients
2 heads	Fresh broccoli
½	Sweet or red onion
1 cup	Shredded cheddar cheese
1 lb	Bacon
1 cup	Miracle Whip
½ cup	Sugar
2 tbsp	Apple cider vinegar

Directions
1. Clean broccoli and chop into bite-sized pieces. Chop onion.
2. Fry bacon until crisp. Drain and crumble.
3. Mix broccoli, onion, bacon, and cheese.
4. Mix Miracle Whip, sugar, and vinegar. Mix into broccoli mix.
5. Can be topped with ¼ cup raisins and/or nuts for more fiber.

*****

Cole Slaw

(from Terry Bradley, 2004 Conference Cookbook)

Ingredients
16 oz. bag shredded cabbage and carrot coleslaw mix
12 oz. bag shredded broccoli, carrot, and red cabbage slaw mix

Dressing

1 to 1½ cups	Mayonnaise (low-calorie or low-fat is fine)
¾ cup	Sour cream (low-fat is fine)
¾ cup	Apple cider vinegar
1 tsp	Garlic powder
2 tsp	Onion powder
1 tsp	Salt (to taste)
½ tsp	Pepper (to taste)

Directions
1. Mix the dressing ingredients together in a large bowl.
2. Add the shredded vegetables and toss well to coat.
3. Keep mixture refrigerated until you are ready to serve.

✳✳✳✳✳

BREADS AND CRACKERS

Banana Nut Muffins

(from Jann Bowne)

Ingredients

½ cup	Butter or margarine, softened
1 cup	Sugar
2 large	Eggs
2 large	Bananas, ripe, mashed
1 tsp	Vanilla
1 cup	Buttermilk
½ cup	Chopped pecans
2 cups	GF flour mix (part bean or sorghum flour)

1 tsp	Salt
½ tsp	Baking powder
½ tsp	Baking soda
1 tsp	Xanthan gum

1 tsp   Salt
1 tsp   Baking powder
½ tsp   Baking soda
1 tsp   Xanthan gum

Directions
1. Preheat oven to 400°F. Grease (or line with muffin papers) 12 muffin pan cups.
2. Beat together butter and sugar at medium speed until light and fluffy.
3. Add eggs, one at a time, beating well after each addition. Beat in bananas until smooth.
4. Mix together dry ingredients.
5. Alternately, stir flour mixture and buttermilk into egg mixture until dry ingredients are just moistened.
6. Stir in nuts and vanilla.
7. Spoon batter into prepared pan, filling half-full. Bake until lightly golden, 15 to 18 minutes.
8. Remove from pan and cool on wire rack.

*****

Biscuit Mix

This can be used for biscuits, but it is also great for waffles, pancakes, impossible pies, and coating chicken or chops for frying.

Ingredients
2 cups   Rice flour (white or brown)
1⅔ cups   Potato starch
⅓ cup   Tapioca starch
3 tsp   Baking powder
2½ tsp   Salt
2 tbsp   Sugar
3 tbsp   Egg substitute
1 cup less 1 tbsp Shortening
½ cup   Dry buttermilk powder (I use soy formula)

Directions
1. In a large bowl, whisk all together except shortening.
2. Cut in shortening, until no lumps appear. Store in the refrigerator until ready to use.

*****

Cheese Crackers

(from Barb Meek, 2004 Conference Cookbook)

Ingredients

2 tbsp	Butter
1	Egg
½ tsp	Salt
⅛ tsp	Pepper
2 cups	Grated sharp cheddar cheese
¾ cup	Rice flour
¼ cup	Potato starch flour
1 tsp	Xanthan gum
	Salt for sprinkling

Directions
1. Preheat oven to 400°F.
2. In a mixer, beat butter until creamy.
3. Add egg, salt, and pepper. Beat until blended.
4. Beat in the cheese until combined.
5. Separately mix the flours and xanthan gum. Add to cheese mixture.
6. Work dough into a ball. If needed to form a ball, add 1 tbsp of water at a time.
7. Do not worry about overworking. (My kids love to help. It is like playing with play dough!)
8. Divide ball in half and place on baking sheet. (Or keep ball together and use a large airbake sheet).
9. Cover the ball with plastic wrap to roll out.
10. The thinner it is rolled out, the crunchier the cracker will be. The thicker it is rolled, the more it will taste like cheese bread.

11. When dough is spread out, sprinkle with salt and cut with pastry wheel. Make into 1-in. squares.
12. Bake 4 to 6 minutes until deep golden.

Note: Fiber can be added by adding 1 to 2 tsp flax seed meal in step 5.

*****

Chocolate, Chocolate Chip Muffins

(*from Beth Sisson, 2004 Conference Cookbook*)
This recipe is *very* high in calories, and it is great to bulk up calories in kids who are trying to gain weight. I also add flax seed meal to add fiber to their diet.

Ingredients

1 stick	Butter or margarine
1¼ cups	Sugar
1	Egg
1½ cup	Gluten-Free Pantry French Bread & Pizza Mix
2¼ tsp	Baking powder
⅛ tsp	Salt
¾ to 1 cup	Milk
1 tbsp	Flax seed meal (optional)
½ cup	Chocolate chips (optional)

Directions
1. Mix butter and sugar until creamy. Add egg.
2. In a separate bowl, mix dry ingredients except chips.
3. Alternately add dry ingredients and milk to sugar mix.
4. Add chocolate chips.
5. Pour into muffin papers.
6. Bake at 350°F for 20 to 25 minutes if using regular-size papers. Bake at 325°F for 15 to 20 minutes if using mini papers.

Note: The mini papers are a great way to get a picky little one to eat them!

*****

Graham Crackers

(from Barb Meek, 2004 Conference Cookbook)

Ingredients

2 cups	GF bean flour mix
1 tsp	Xanthan gum
1½ tsp	Salt
1 tsp	Cinnamon
2½ tsp	Baking powder
¾ cup	Butter or margarine
¼ cup	Honey
1 cup	Brown sugar
1 tsp	Vanilla
1 to 2 tbsp	Water
	Cornstarch for rolling

Directions
1. Whisk together dry ingredients and set aside.
2. In a large bowl, beat remaining ingredients except water.
3. Add dry ingredients alternately with water, using just enough to hold the batter in a dough ball that will handle easily.
4. Refrigerate for at least one hour.
5. Preheat oven to 325°F.
6. Lightly grease two 12 in. × 15 in. baking sheets.
7. Using half the dough, work in some cornstarch if necessary to get a ball that is not sticky.
8. Roll out on a cornstarch-dusted piece of plastic wrap to a rectangle 13-in. long.
9. Transfer to a prepared baking sheet by placing a sheet over the dough and flipping the dough onto a baking sheet.
10. Continue rolling out the dough until it completely covers the baking sheet and is about ⅛-in. thick.

11. Cut with pastry wheel.
12. Prick with a fork a couple of times.
13. Bake for about 30 minutes, removing crackers around
    the edge if they get too brown.

Note: Fiber can be added by adding 1 to 2 tsp flax seed meal.

*****

Sandwich Buns

Ingredients

2 cups	Rice flour
1 cup	Tapioca flour
1 cup	Potato starch
2 tsp	Sugar
3½ tsp	Xanthan gum
1½ tbsp	Clear gel* (optional)
⅔ cup	Dry milk powder (for lactose intolerance use soy baby formula)
1½ tsp	Salt
3	Large eggs
½ stick	Butter or margarine
1¼ cup	Water
1 tsp	Vinegar
1¾ cups	Warm water (110–115°F)
¼ cup plus 2 tsp	Sugar
2 packs	Rapid rise dry yeast

Directions
1. Combine flours, sugar, xanthan gum, clear gel,
   milk powder, and salt in a large bowl of a heavy
   duty mixer.
2. In a large measuring cup, cover eggs with warm
   water and allow to stand.
3. Warm butter in vinegar and 1¼ cups warm water.

4. In a measuring cup, stir together the remaining ½ cup warm water, 2 tsp sugar, and yeast. Let stand until yeast foams slightly.

5. At low speed, blend the dry ingredients. Pour in the shortening mixture, blend, then add the eggs. Blend, then add the dissolved yeast. Beat at highest speed for two to three minutes. The dough will be very sticky.

6. Spray muffin top baking pans with cooking spray. Using slightly wet hands, pat the dough gently until you reach the edges of the circle. Allow the dough to rise in a warm place. When doubled, bake at 350°F for 20 to 25 minutes.

7. *Pizza Crusts*: This recipe can also be used to bake pizza shells. Brush the dough lightly with olive oil to seal the surface before baking. The shells take about eight minutes at 400°F.

*Clear gel is a generic gelatin available in some grocery stores.

*****

Soft White Bread

(from Irene Edge, 2004 Conference Cookbook)

Ingredients

Sift together

2 cups	White rice flour
2 cups	Tapioca flour
4 tsp	Xanthan gum
¼ cup	Sugar
⅔ cup	Dry milk
1 tsp	Salt

Stir in:

| 4 tsp | Active dry yeast (2 pkg) |

Separately combine:

3	Eggs, beaten
2 cups	Water
4 tbsp	Margarine, melted
1 tsp	Vinegar

Directions
1. Mix all ingredients together.
2. Let dough rise in bowl.
3. Pour into greased bread pans and let dough rise.
4. Bake at 350°F for 20 to 25 minutes.

Tip: For pizza: Bake 12 minutes. Add toppings. Bake additional 15 minutes.

Potato pizza: Bake crust. Melt 4 tsp margarine, add ½ tsp garlic. Spread over crust. Layer with sliced white potatoes (can be canned). Cover with Colby cheddar cheese. Sprinkle with bacon (cooked, cooled, and crumbled) and diced onions. Bake 15 minutes.

✳✳✳✳✳

West Tennessee Corn Bread

(from Brenda Lucas, 2002 Conference Cookbook)

Ingredients
1	Egg
¼ cup	Mayonnaise (do *not* use reduced-fat or fat-free)
¼ cup	Buttermilk
1 tbsp	Oil
1 cup	Yellow corn meal
¼ cup	Sugar
1½ tsp	Baking powder
¼ tsp	Salt

Directions
1. In a bowl, beat first four ingredients until smooth.
2. Combine remaining ingredients and add to egg mixture.
3. Place in greased and dusted (with cornmeal) oven-proof 6-in. skillet or round baking dish.
4. Bake at 425°F for 18 to 20 minutes.

✳✳✳✳✳

COOKIES AND DESSERTS

Angel Pie

(from Sandy Robbins)
Serves 8

Ingredients
Meringue

4	Egg whites
¼ tsp	Cream of tartar
1 cup	Sugar
	Pinch of salt
1 tsp	Vanilla

Filling

4	Egg yolks
½ cup	Sugar
⅓ cup	Lemon juice
2 tbsp	Grated lemon peel
2 cups	Whipping cream (whipped)
	Toasted almonds (for garnish)

To make the meringue:

Directions
1. Preheat oven to 275°F.
2. Beat egg whites until frothy.
3. Add cream of tartar and beat until stiff, gradually adding sugar and salt.
4. Fold in vanilla. Spread in a 9-in. buttered pie pan covering bottom and sides.

5. Shape with the back of a spoon, making the bottom ¼-in. thick and the sides 1-in. thick.
6. Bake for one hour; leave in the oven to cool for 1 hour.

To make the filling:

1. Beat egg yolks until lemon-colored, gradually adding sugar, lemon juice, and lemon peel.
2. Cook in the top of a double boiler over hot water (not touching pan) until thick, stirring constantly. This will take between five and eight minutes. Cool until room temperature.
3. Fold in 1 cup of cream, whipped. Spread over meringue and cover with 1 cup of cream, whipped. Sprinkle toasted almonds over the top.
4. Refrigerate a minimum of 12 hours. May be made the day before serving.

Note: You can "cheat" and use Cool Whip instead of freshly whipped cream, but it might not be as good!

*****

Buckeyes in Winter

(from Sylvia Bower and Jessica Turner)

Dough
1½ cups	GF flour
1 tsp	Xanthan gum
½ tsp	Salt
½ cup	Unsweetened cocoa
½ tsp	Baking soda
½ cup	White sugar
½ cup	Brown sugar
½ cup	Butter (one stick)
¼ cup	Creamy peanut butter
1 tsp	Vanilla
1	Egg

Filling

¾ cup	Creamy peanut butter
¾ cup	Powdered sugar

Instructions

1. Preheat oven to 375°F.
2. In a small bowl combine flour, xanthan gum, salt, cocoa, and baking soda. Blend well and set aside. (Or mix in a tightly sealed plastic bag.)
3. In a large mixing bowl, beat the sugars, butter, and peanut butter until light and fluffy.
4. Add vanilla and egg, beating well.
5. Stir in flour mixture until blended. Refrigerate while making filling.
6. In a small bowl, combine peanut butter and powdered sugar and blend well.
7. Using your hands, form twenty 1- to 2-in. balls of the filling (they expand while baking).
8. To make the buckeyes, shape 1 tsp of dough into a round flat patty.
9. Place a ball of filling in the center and ease the dough around it, covering it, but leaving a small opening to resemble a buckeye.
10. Bake at 375°F for seven to nine minutes until set.
11. Remove immediately and roll in powdered sugar.

Yield: About 20 cookies.

*****

Deluxe Buckwheat Almond Cake

(*from Sherry Weinstein; reprinted with permission from* The Birkett Mills Buckwheat Cookbook, *The Birkett Mills, Penn Yan, NY*)

Ingredients

1½ cups	Sliced almonds, with skin on
¾ cup	Unsalted butter, softened
¾ cup	Sugar, divided
4	Eggs, separated

⅛ tsp	Salt
2 tsp	Vanilla extract
½ cup	Light buckwheat flour
½ cup	Raspberry preserves
10-in.	round paper doily
1 tbsp	Confectioners' sugar

Instructions
1. Oil bottom of 9 in. × 1½ in. round cake pan and line with wax paper.
2. Finely grind almonds in food processor, blender, or nut-chopper.
3. In large bowl, cream butter and 6 tbsp sugar. Beat in yolks, one at a time. Stir in vanilla and almonds.
4. In medium bowl, beat egg whites and salt to soft peaks; gradually add remaining sugar, beating until soft, glossy peaks form.
5. Lightly fold one-fourth of the beaten whites into the batter. Sift one-fourth of the flour over batter; combine lightly. Alternately add remaining whites and flour in this manner.
6. Pour batter into pan. Bake at 350°F for 30 minutes or until tester inserted into center comes out clean.
7. Cool on rack 10 minutes; remove from pan.
8. When cool, slice horizontally into two layers. Place bottom layer, cut side up, on plate; spread with preserves. Top with remaining layer, cut side down.
9. Place doily on top; sprinkle with confectioner's sugar; remove doily.

✳✳✳✳✳

Easy Flourless Chocolate Cake

(from Sylvia Bower)

Ingredients
| ½ cup | Unsalted butter |

¾ cup	Sugar
3	Eggs
4 oz	Bittersweet chocolate
½ cup	Unsweetened cocoa

Ganache (*recipe follows*)
Serve with whipped cream

Instructions:
Cake:

1. Preheat oven to 375°F. Grease an 8-in. round pan.
2. In a double boiler over barely simmering water, melt chocolate and butter until smooth. Remove from heat and whisk in sugar.
3. Add eggs and combine well.
4. Sift in cocoa powder and whisk until smooth.
5. Pour batter into prepared pan. Bake for about 25 minutes or until thin crust is formed. Cool cake for five minutes before removing from pan to cool completely on rack. Transfer to serving plate and dust lightly with cocoa powder or spread with ganache (recipe follows). Refrigerate.

Ganache

¼ cup	Heavy cream
2 tbsp	Unsalted butter
4 oz.	Semisweet chocolate, chopped or chips

In a small pan, bring the cream and butter to a simmer. Remove from heat, add chocolate, and stir until smooth.

*****

Easy Fruit Salad

(from Diane Lott)

Ingredients
1 can   Lite chunky mixed fruit

1 can	Pineapple tidbits or chunks in natural juice
1 pkg (12–16 oz.)	Frozen strawberries, thawed
2	Bananas, sliced

Chill canned fruit. Mix together with thawed strawberries and bananas. Serve chilled.

*****

Fruit Fluff

(from Stephanie Olson, 2004 Conference Cookbook)

Ingredients
8 oz.	Cool Whip
1 pkg	GF vanilla pudding, small
¾ cup	Milk (or soy milk)
1 can	Mandarin oranges, drained
2	Bananas, sliced

Directions
1. Whip together the Cool Whip, pudding, and milk for a base.
2. Fold in the fruit.

Tip: Any fruits can be substituted for the bananas and oranges. Try strawberries, grapes, pineapple, or any other fruit that "tickles your fancy."

*****

Million Dollar Salad

(from Elizabeth Sager, 2002 Conference Cookbook)

Ingredients
1 can	Sweetened condensed milk
½ cup	Lemon juice
20 oz.	can Crushed pineapple, well-drained
1 cup	Coconut

| 1 cup | Chopped pecans |
| 1 large tub | Cool Whip |

Directions
1. Combine milk with lemon juice; add remaining ingredients. Delicious!

*****

Minute Chocolate Mug Cake

Makes one cake but it is enough for two if you want to share.

Ingredients

1	Coffee mug
4 tbsp	GF flour
4 tbsp	Sugar
2 tbsp	Baking cocoa
Dash	Xanthan gum
1	Egg
3 tbsp	Milk
3 tbsp	Oil
3 tbsp	Chocolate chips
1 tbsp	Chopped nuts (optional)
¼ tsp	Vanilla

Directions
1. Add dry ingredients to mug and mix well.
2. Add the egg and mix thoroughly.
3. Pour in the milk and oil and mix well.
4. Add the chocolate chips and vanilla, and mix again.
5. Put the mug in the microwave for three minutes on high. The cake will rise over the top of the mug, but do not be alarmed! Allow to cool, and tip out onto a plate.

*****

Peanut Butter Fudge

(from Judy Hamill)

Ingredients

4 cups	Sugar
1 jar	Smooth peanut butter
½ cup	Butter
1 pint	Marshmallow cream
1 tsp	Vanilla
1 can	Evaporated milk

Directions
1. Combine sugar, butter, and milk in heavy pan and stir constantly until it comes to a full boil.
2. Reduce heat and continue stirring for seven minutes.
3. Remove from heat.
4. With mixer on low or by hand, stir in peanut butter, marshmallow cream, and vanilla. When the mixture is not shiny, spread immediately on a buttered jelly roll pan.
5. Cut when cool.

*****

Sample Weekly Menu—Breakfast

Sunday	Monday	Tuesday	Wednesday	Thursday	Friday	Saturday
Breakfast pizza Sliced fruit Milk	Hot cereal (GF oatmeal or cream Of rice cereal or cream of buckwheat mixed with nuts, raisins, and ground flax seed) Milk	Yogurt fruit smoothie GF cereal bar	Chex cereal topped with banana and 1–2 tbsp GF granola Milk Orange juice	Breakfast wrap—Eggs-scrambled with green pepper, onions and cheese and 1 tbsp salsa wrapped in a GF corn or GF flour tortilla Sliced orange	Gluten free waffles topped with sliced strawberries and blueberries Milk	Yogurt parfait-vanilla yogurt layered with gluten-free granola & berries of choice

Sample Weekly Menu—Lunch

Sunday	Monday	Tuesday	Wednesday	Thursday	Friday	Saturday
Chef salad	GF "lunchable"	Tortilla soup	GF vegetable soup	Baked potato topped with chili and cheese	Banana nut muffin	Tacos
GF corn-bread	Sliced lunchmeat and cheese	GF tortilla chips	GF crackers	Sliced apples	Tuna salad	2 corn tortillas stuffed with
Mixed fruit	GF whole grain crackers	Grilled ham and cheese on GF bread	Peanut butter		Baby carrots	ground beef seasoned with
	Baby carrots	Fresh fruit	Fresh fruit		String cheese	GF taco seasoning and
	Grapes				Fresh fruit	onions, lettuce, tomato, cheese and salsa
	GF pudding cup					Pears
						Black bean and corn salad

Sample Weekly Menu—Dinner

Sunday	Monday	Tuesday	Wednesday	Thursday	Friday	Saturday
Oven baked chicken	Gluten-free pizza	Turkey kielbasa with potatoes and peppers	Pork chop topped with peach salsa and 1 tsp mustard	Impossible chicken and broccoli pie	Rice bowl 1 cup cooked brown rice topped with stir fried chicken and vegetables	Spaghetti squash with spaghetti sauce
Mashed potatoes	Tossed salad	Easy fruit salad	Corn pancakes	Mixed fruit	Sliced pineapple	Tossed green salad
Broccoli salad	Applesauce		Green beans			Mandarin oranges
Sliced peaches						

Resources

Mary Kay Sharrett

General

Acceptability of Foods and Food Ingredients for the Gluten-Free Diet Pocket Dictionary
Canadian Celiac Association

American Dietetic Association Easy Gluten-Free: Expert Nutrition Advice with More Than 100 Recipes
Tricia Thompson MS, RD and Marlisa Brown, MS, RD, CDE, CDN

Celiac Disease: A Hidden Epidemic
Peter Green, MD, and Rory Jones

Celiac Disease for Dummies
Ian Blumer, MD, and Sheila Crowe, MD

Celiac Disease Nutrition Guide, 3rd Edition
Tricia Thompson, MS, RD

The Academy of Nutrition and Dietetics
www.eatright.org

A Clinical Guide to Gluten-Related Disorders
Edited by Alessio Fasano, MD.

The Complete Idiot's Guide to Gluten-Free Eating
Eve Adamson and Tricia Thompson, MS, RD

The Essential Gluten-Free Restaurant Guide
Triumph Dining

Gluten-Free Diet: A Comprehensive Resource Guide
Shelley Case

Gluten-Free Hassle-Free: A Simple, Sane, Dietitian-Approved
   Program for Eating Your Way Back to Health, Second Edition
Marlisa Brown, MS, RD, CDE, CDN

Gluten Freedom: The Nation's Leading Expert Offers the Essen-
   tial Guide to a Healthy, Gluten-Free Lifestyle
Alessio Fasano, MD, and Susie Flaherty

Kids with Celiac Disease: A Family Guide to Raising Happy,
   Healthy, Gluten-Free Children
Danna Korn

Real Life with Celiac Disease: Troubleshooting and Thriving
   Gluten Free
Melinda Dennis, MS, RD, LDN, and Daniel Leffler, MD, MS

What Nurses Know… Gluten-Free Lifestyle
Sylvia Llewelyn Bower, RN

The Ultimate Guide to Gluten-Free Living
Celiac Disease Center at Columbia University

Let's Eat Out Around the World Gluten Free and Allergy Free,
   Fourth Edition
Kim Koeller and Robert La France

Books for GF Kids

Bagels, Buddy and Me
Written and illustrated by Melanie Krumrey

*Beyond Rice Cakes: A Young Person's Guide to Cooking, Eating
    & Living Gluten-Free*
Vanessa Martin

Eating Gluten-Free with Emily
Bonnie J. Kruszka, Illustrated by Richard S. Cihlar

The Gluten-Free Kid. A Celiac Disease Survival Guide
Melissa London

The Gluten Glitch
Stacie John

How I Eat Without Wheat
Karen Fine, Illustrated by Russ Novak

*Lunch with Quinn: The Story of One Child's Diagnosis and
    Management of Celiac Disease*
Angela Porter

No More Cupcakes and Tummy Aches
Jax Peters Lowell, Illustrated by Jane Kirkwood

The Trouble That Jack Had
Jane Pintavalle and Diane Pintavalle

Cookbooks

The Gluten-Free Gourmet
More from the Gluten-Free Gourmet
The Gluten-Free Gourmet Cooks Fast and Healthy
*The Gluten-Free Gourmet Bakes Bread: More than 200 Wheat-
    Free Recipes*
The Gluten-Free Gourmet Makes Dessert
Gluten-Free Comfort Foods
Bette Hagman

Gluten-Free 101
125 Gluten-Free Vegetarian Recipes
*Gluten-Free Quick & Easy—From Prep to Plate without the
    Fuss: 200+ Recipes for People with Food Sensitivities*
1000 Gluten-Free Recipes
100 Best Gluten-Free Recipes
*Cooking Free: 200+ Flavorful Recipes for People with Food
    Allergies and Multiple Food Sensitivities*
Carol Fenster, PhD

Incredible Edible Gluten-Free Food for Kids
Sheri L Sanderson

The Wheat-Free Gluten-Free Dessert Cookbook
Wheat-Free Gluten-Free Cookbook for Kids & Busy Adults
The Wheat-Free Gluten-Free Reduced Calorie Cookbook
Wheat-Free Gluten-Free Cookbook for Special Diets
Connie Sarros

GluTEEN Free: A Cookbook for Teens
Cody Ankerman

Pulses and the Gluten-Free Diet
www.pulsecanada.com/pulses-and-the-gluten-free-diet

Nearly Normal Cooking for Gluten-Free Eating
Jules E.D. Shepard

Gluten-Free Baking Classics: 100 Recipes for the Breads,
    Pastries and Pizzas You Love to Eat
Annalise G. Roberts and Peter Green

You Won't Believe It Is Gluten-Free: 500 Gluten-Free Delicious
    Recipes for Healthy Living
Gluten-Free. Kitchen: Over 135 Delicious Recipes for People
    with Gluten Intolerance or Wheat Allergy
Roben Ryberg

Delicious Breads: Wheat Free and Gluten Free
Lynn Rae Reis

Gluten-Free Every Day Cookbook: More than 100 Easy and
    Delicious Recipes from the Gluten-Free Chef
Robert Landolphi

Make It Fast, Cook It Slow: The Big Book of Everyday Slow
    Cooking
Stephanie O'Dea

Magazines

Allergic Living Magazine
www.allergicliving.com

Bob and Ruth's Dining and Travel Club
www.bobandruths.com

Delight Gluten Free
www.delightgfmagazine.com

Easy Eats
www.easyeats.com

Gluten-Free Living Magazine
www.glutenfreeliving.com

Living Without Magazine
www.livingwithout.com

Scott Free Newsletter
www.celiac.com

Simply Gluten Free Magazine
www.simplyglutenfreemag.com

Websites

General

Celiac Discussion List Archives
CELIAC-subscribe-request@LISTSERV.ICORS.ORG

Celiac Disease Awareness Campaign National Institutes of Health
http://celiac.nih.gov

Celiac Disease and Food Sensitivities
www.livebetteramerica.com/health-nutrition/celiac-food-sensitivities

Celiac Now
www.CeliacNow.org

Celiac Organization
www.celiac.com

The Celiac Scene
www.theceliacscene.com

Gastro Kids
www.gastrokids.org

Gluten Free
www.Glutenfree.com

The Gluten-Free Dietitian
www.glutenfreedietitian.com

Gluten-Free Restaurant Awareness Program
www.gluten.net/gfrap

Gluten-Free Watch Dog
www.glutenfreewatchdog.org

National Digestive Diseases Clearinghouse
www.niddk.nih.gov/health/digest/pubs/celiac/index.htm

National Institutes of Health Consensus Conference on Celiac
  Disease
http://consensus.nih.gov/2004/2004celiacdisease118html.htm

R.O.C.K Raising Our Celiac Kids
www.celiackids.com

Steve Plogsted, Pharm.D, Medication list
www.glutenfreedrugs.com

Celiac Research Centers

Celiac Disease Center at Nationwide Children's Hospital
www.nationwidechildrens.org/celiac-disease

Celiac Center at Beth Israel Deaconess Medical Center,
  Massachusetts
www.bidmc.org/celiaccenter

Celiac Disease Center at Columbia University
www.celiacdiseasecenter.org

Celiac Disease Clinic at Mayo Clinic, Minnesota
www.mayoclinic.org/celiac-disease

Center for Celiac Research at MassGeneral Hospital for Children
www.celiaccenter.org

University of Chicago Celiac Disease Program
www.celiacdisease.net

University of Virginia Health System
www.healthsystem.virginia.edu/internet/digestive-
  health/nutrition/celiacsupport.cfm

National Resource Groups

American Celiac Disease Alliance
www.americanceliac.org

Canadian Celiac Association
Mississauga, ON
www.celiac.ca

Celiac Disease Foundation
Studio City, CA
www.celiac.org

Celiac Sprue Association
Omaha, NE
www.csaceliacs.org

Gluten Intolerance Group of WA
Auburn, WA
www.gluten.net

National Foundation for Celiac Awareness
www.celiaccentral.org

Gluten Free Companies

1-2-3 Gluten-Free, Inc
www.123glutenfree.com

Against the Grain Gourmet
www.againstthegraingourmet.com

Amy's Kitchen
www.amyskitchen.com

Ancient Harvest Quinoa Corporation
www.quinoa.net

Andean Dreams
www.andeandreams.com

Around the World Gourmet
www.aroundtheworldgourmet.com

Authentic Foods
www.authenticfoods.com

Baby Cakes Bakery NYC
www.babycakesnyc.com

Bakery on Main
www.bakeryonmain.com

Bloomfield Farms/Blendpak
www.bloomfieldfarmsstore.com

Blue Diamond Growers
www.bluediamond.com

Bob's Red Mill Natural Foods, Inc.
www.bobsredmill.com

Breads from Anna
www.breadsfromanna.com

Celiac Specialties
www.celiacspecialties.com

Celinal Foods
www.celinalfoods.com

Chebe Bread
www.chebe.com

Cherrybrook Kitchen
www.cherrybrookkitchen.com

Edward and Sons
www.edwardandsons.com

Ener-G Foods, Inc.
www.ener-g.com

Enjoy Life Foods
www.enjoylifefoods.com

Food for Life Baking Company
www.food-for-life.com

French Meadow Bakery
www.frenchmeadow.com

General Mills Gluten-Free Products
www.bettycrocker.com/products/gluten-free-products

GF Harvest
www.glutenfreeoats.com

The Gluten-Free Mall
www.glutenfreemall.com

The Gluten-Free Trading Company
www.glutenfree.net

Gluten Freeda
www.glutenfreeda.com

Gluten Solutions
www.glutensolutions.com

Glutino
www.glutino.com

Go Picnic
www.gopicnic.com

Goodbye Gluten
www.goodbyeglutenbakeries.com

Jules Gluten Free Flours and Baking Mixes
www.julesglutenfree.com

Katz Bakery
www.katzglutenfree.com

Kettle Cuisine
www.kettlecuisine.com

Kingsmill Food
www.kingsmillfoods.com

Kinnikinnick Foods, Inc.
www.kinnikinnick.com

Lundberg Family Farms
www.lundberg.com

Maple Grove Foods
www.maplegrovefoods.com

Mary's Gone Crackers
www.marysgonecrackers.com

Mr. Ritt's Bakery
www.mrritts.com

Mrs. Leepers
www.mrsleepers.com

Namaste Foods
www.namastefoods.com

Nature's Path
www.naturespath.com

Nu-World Foods
www.nuworldfoods.com

Pamela's Products
www.pamelasproducts.com

Rizopia Food Products, Inc.
www.rizopia.com

Rudi's
www.rudisbakery.com

Schär
www.schar.com

Snyders of Hanover
www.snydersofhanover.com

TH Foods
www.thfoods.com

Tinkyada
www.tinkyada.com

Udi's
www.udisglutenfree.com

Vans Natural Foods
www.vansfoods.com/our-products-all-gluten-free

Gluten Free Oats

Cream Hill Estates
www.creamhillestates.com

GF Harvest
www.glutenfreeoats.com

Only Oats by Farm Pure Foods
www.onlyoats.com

Bibliography

Addolorato, G., Capristo, E., Ghittoni, G., Valeri, C., Masciana, R., Ancona, C., & Gasbarrini G. (2001). "Anxiety but not depression decreases in coeliac patients after one-year gluten-free diet: a longitudinal study." *Scandinavian Journal of Gastroenterology, 36*(5), 502–506.

Addolorato, G., Diguida, D., De Rossi, G., Valenza, V., Domenicali, M., Caputo, F., ..., Gasbarrini, G. (2004). "Regional cerebral hypoperfusion in patients with celiac disease." *American Journal of Medicine, 116*(5), 312–317.

Agardh, D., Nilsson, A., Tuomi, T., Linberg, B., Carlsson, A. K., Lernmark, A., & Ivarsson, S. A. (2001). "Prediction of silent celiac disease at diagnosis of childhood type I diabetes by tissue transglutaminase autoantibodies and HLA." *Pediatric Diabetes, 2*(2), 58–65.

Armstrong, M. J., Hegade, V. S, & Robins, G. (2012). "Advances in coeliac disease." *Current Opinion in Gastroenterology, 28*(2), 104–112. doi: 10.1097/MOG.0b013e32834d0844.

Assiri, A., Saeed, A., Al Sarkhy, A., El Mousan, M. I., & El Matary, W. (2013). "Celiac disease presenting as rickets in Saudi children." *Annals of Saudi Medicine, 33*(1), 49–51.

Aziz, I., & Sanders, D. S. (2012). "Emerging concepts: from coeliac disease to non-celiac gluten sensitivity." *The Proceedings of the Nutrition Society, 71*(4), 576–580. doi: 10.1017/S002966511200081X.

Barrett, J. S., & Gibson, P. R. (2012). "Fermentable oligosaccharides, disaccharides, monosaccharides and polyols (FODMAPS) and nonallergic food intolerance: FODMAPS or food chemicals?" *Therapeutic Advances in Gastroenterology, 5*(4), 261–268. doi: 10.1177/1756283X11436241.

Bhutani, J., Bhutani, S., & Kumai, J. (2013). "Patient-centric care: managing celiac disease." *Indian Journal of Endocrinology and Metabolism, 17*(1), 177.

Biesiekierski, J. R., Peters, S. L., Newnham, E. D., Rosella, O., Muir, J. G., & Gibson, P. R. (2013). "No effects of gluten in patients with self-reported non-celiac gluten sensitivity after dietary reduction of fermentable, poorly absorbed, short-chain carbohydrates." *Gastroenterology, 145*(2), 320-8.e1–320-8.e3. doi: .1053/j.gastro.2013.04.051.

Book, L., Hart, A., Black, J., Feolo, M., Zone, J. J., & Neuhausen, S. L. (2001). "Prevalence and clinical characteristics of celiac disease in Down syndrome in a US study." *American Journal of Medical Genetics, 98*(1), 70–74.

Bower, S. (2011). *What Nurses Know...Gluten-Free Lifestyle.* New York, NY: Demos Health: 18–23, 75, 76, 149–150.

Brown, W. R., & Tayal, S. (2013). "Microscopic colitis. A review." *Journal of Digestive Diseases, 14*(6), 277–281. doi: 10.1111/1751-2980.12046.

Bucci, C., Zingone, F., Russo, I., Morra, I., Tortora, R., Pogna, N., ..., Ciacca C. (2013). "Gliadin does not induce mucosal inflammation or basophil activation in patients with nonceliac gluten sensitivity." *Clinical Gastroenterology and Hepatology, 11*(10), 1294–1299.e1. doi: 10.1016/j.cgh.2013.04.022.

Buie, T. (2013). "The relationship of autism and gluten." *Clinical Therapeutics, 35*(5), 578–583. doi: 10.1016/jclinthera.2013.04.011.

Bushara, K. O. (2005). "Neurological presentation of celiac disease." *Gastroenterology, 128*(4 Suppl 1), S92–S97.

Carta, M. G., Hardoy, M. C., Boi. M. F., Mariotti, S., Carpiniello, B., & Usai, P. (2002). "Association between panic disorder, major depressive disorder, and celiac disease: possible role of thyroid autoimmunity." *Journal Psychosomatic Research, 53*(3), 789–793.

Carta, M. G., Hardoy, M. C., Usai, P., Carpiniello, B., & Angst J. (2003). "Recurrent brief depression in celiac disease." *Journal of Psychosomatic Research, 55*(6), 573–574.

Chmielewska, A., Szajewska, H., & Shamir, R. (2013). "Celiac disease: prevention strategies through early infant nutrition." *World Review of Nutrition and Dietetic, 108*, 91–97. doi: 0.1159/000351491.

Chopra, D., & Tanzi, R. (2012). *Super Brain.* New York, NY: Harmony Books.

Ciacca, C., Iavarone, A., Siniscalchi, M., Romano, R., & DeRosa A. (2002). "Psychological dimensions of celiac disease: toward an integrated approach." *Digestive Diseases and Sciences, 47*(9), 2082–2087.

DeMaristris, L., Picardi, A., Siniscalco, D., Riccio, M. P., Sapone, A., Cariello, R., ..., Bravaccio C. (2013). "Antibodies against food antigens in patients with autistic spectrum disorders." *BioMed Research International, 2013*, 729349. doi:10.1155/2013/729349.

DiGiacomo, D. V., Tennyson, C. A., Green, P. H., & Demmer, R. T. (2013). "Prevalence of gluten-free diet adherence among individuals without celiac disease in the USA: results from the Continuous National Health and Nutrition Examination Survey 2009–2010." *Scandinavian Journal of Gastroenterology, 48*(8), 921–925. doi: 10.3109/00365521.2013.809598.

Duggan, J. M. (2004). "Coeliac disease: the great imitator." *Medical Journal of Australia,* May 17; 180 (10), 524–526.

Fouda, M. A., Khan, A. A., Sultan, M. S., Rios, L. P., McAssey, K., & Armstrong, D. (2012). "Evaluation and management of skeletal health in celiac disease: position statement." *Canadian Journal of Gastroenterology, 26*(11), 819–829.

Freeman, H. J. (2004). "Strongly positive tissue transglutaminase antibody assays without celiac disease." *Canadian Journal of Gastroenterology, 18*(1), 25–28.

Gasbarrini, G., Miele, L., Corazza, G., & Gasbarrini, A. (2010). "When was celiac disease born?: the Italian case from the Archeologic Site of Cosa." *Journal of Clinical Gastroenterology, 44*(7), 502–503.

Green, P. H., & Jabri, B. (2003). "Celiac disease." *The Lancet, 362*(9381), 383–391.

Green, P. H., Jabri, B. (2002). "Celiac disease and other precursors to small-bowel malignancy." *Gastroenterology Clinics of North America, 31*(2), 625–639.

Green, P.H., & Jones, R. (2005). *Celiac Disease: A Hidden Epidemic*. New York, NY: HarperCollins.

Green, P. H., & Pampertab, S. D. (2004). "Small bowel carcinoma and celiac disease." *Gut, 53*(5), 774.

Green, P. H., Rostami, K., & Marsh, M. N. (2005). "Diagnosis of coeliac disease." *Best Practice and Research Clinical Gastroenterology, 19*(3), 389–400.

Gudjonsdotter, A. H., Nilsson, S., Ek, J., Kristiansson, B., & Ascher, H. (2004). "The risk of celiac disease in with at least two affected siblings." *Journal of Pediatric Gastroenterology Nutrition, 38*(3), 338–342.

Hadjivassiliou, M., Aeschlimann, P., Sander, D. S., Maki, M., Kaukinen, K., Grunewald, R. A, ..., Aeschlimann, D. P. (2013). "Transglutaminase 6 antibodies in the diagnosis of gluten ataxia." *Neurology, 80*(19), 1740–1745. doi: 10.1212/WNL.0b013e3182919070. Epub 2013 Apr 10.

Haskinson, S., Colditz, G., Manson, J., & Speizer, F. editors. (2001). *Healthy Women, Healthy Lives: A Guide to Preventing Disease, from the Landmark Nurses, Health Study*. New York, NY: Simon and Schuster.

Hoffenberg, E. J., MacKenzie, T., Barriga, K. J., Eisenbarth, G. S. Bao, F., Haas, J. E., ..., Norris, J. M. (2003). "A prospective study of the incidence of childhood celiac disease." *Journal of Pediatrics. 143*(3), 308–314.

Ivarsson, A., Myléus, A., Norström, F., van der Pals, M., Rosén, A., Högberg, L., ..., Stenhammar, L. (2013). "Prevalence of childhood celiac disease and infant feeding." *Pediatrics. 131*(3): e687–e694. doi: 10.1542/peds.2012-1015.

Lau, N. M., Green, P. H., Taylor, A. K., Hellberg, D., Ajamian, M., Tan, C. Z., ..., Alaedini, A. (2013). "Markers of celiac disease and gluten sensitivity in children with autism." *PLoS One, 8*(6), e66155.

Leffler, D., Saha, S., & Farrell, R. J. (2003). "Celiac disease." *The American Journal of Managed Care, 9*(12), 825–831.

Lepers, S., Couignoux, S., Colombel, J. F., & Dubucquoi, S. (2004). "Celiac disease in adults: new aspects." *La Revue de Medicine Interne, 25*(1), 22–34.

Ludvigsson, J. F, & Fasano, A. (2012). "Timing of introduction of gluten and celiac disease risk." *Annals of Nutrition and Metabolism, 60*(Suppl 2), 22–29. doi: 10.1159/000335335.

Lundin, K. E., & Alaedini, A. (2012). "Non-celiac gluten sensitivity." *Gastrointestinal Endoscopy Clinics of North America, 22*(4), 723–734. doi: 10.1016/j.giec.2012.07.006.

Machado, A. P., Silva, L. R., Zausner, B., Oliverira Jde, A., Diniz, D. R., & de Oliveira, J. (2013). "Undiagnosed celiac disease in women with infertility." *The Journal of Reproductive Medicine, 58*(1–2), 61–66.

Malamut, G., & Cellier C. (2013). "Refractory coeliac disease." *Current Opinion Oncology, 25*(5), 445–451.

Malamut, G., Murray, J. A., & Cellier C. (2012). "Refractory celiac disease." *Gastrointestinal Endoscopy Clinics of North America, 22*(4), 759–772. doi: 10.1016/j.giec.2012.07.007.

Matthews, D. A. (1998). *The Faith Factor: Proof of the Healing Power of Prayer.* New York, NY: Penguin.

Mendes, F. B., Hissa-Elian, A., Abreu, M. A., & Goncalves, V. S. (2013). "Review: dermatitis herpetiformis." *Anais Brasileiros de Dermatologia, 88*(4), 594–599. doi: 10.1590/abd1806-4841.20131775.

Milewicz, T., Pulka, M., Galicka-Latala, D., Rzepka, E., & Krzvisiek, J. (2011). "Sprue-coeliac disease and fertility." *Przegląd Lekarski, 68*(9), 641–644. Review. Polish.

Mooney, P. D., Aziz, I., & Sanders, D. S. (2013). "Non-celiac gluten sensitivity: clinical relevance and recommendations for future research." *Neurogastroenterology Motility, 25*(11), 864–871. doi: 10.1111/nmo.12216.

Murray, J. A., Watson, T., Clearman, B., & Mitros, F. (2004). "Effect of a gluten-free diet on gastrointestinal symptoms in celiac disease." *American Journal of Clinical Nutrition, 79*(4), 669–673.

Moreno, M. L., Vazquez, H., Mazure, R., Smecuol, E., Niveloni, S., Pedreire, S., ..., Bai, J. C. (2004). "Stratification of bone fracture risk in patients with celiac disease." *Clinical Gastroenterology/Hepatology, 2* (2), 127–134.

National Institutes of Health, National Institute of Diabetes and Digestive and Kidney Diseases, Celiac Disease. (2013). Retrieved from www.digestive.niddk.nih.gov/diseases/pubs/celiac.

"The New Medicine," PBS Documentary, shown April 6, 2006. Directed by Muffie Meyer.

Parakkal, D., Du, H., Semer, R., Ehernpreis, E. D., & Guandalini, S. (2012). "Do gastroenterologists adhere to diagnostic and treatment guidelines for celiac disease?" *Journal Clinical Gastroenterology, 46*(2), e12–e20. doi: 10.1097/MCG.0b013e31822f0da0.

Petroniene, R., Dubcenco, E., Baker, J. P., Ottaway, C. A., Tang, S. J., Zanati, S. A., ..., Jeejeebhoy, K. N. (2005). "Given capsule endoscopy in celiac disease." *American Journal of Gastroenterology, 100* (3), 685–694.

Philip, R., Patidar, P., Saran, S., Agarwal, P., Arva, T., & Gupta, K. (2012). "Endocrine manifestations of celiac disease." *Indian Journal of Endocrinology and Metabolism*, *16*(Suppl 2), S506–S508. doi: 10.4103/2230-8210.104149.

Potocki, P., & Hozyasz, K. (2002). "Psychiatric symptoms and coeliac disease." *Psychiatria Polska [Psychiatr Pol]*, *36*(4), 567–578.

Riddle, M. S., Murray, J. A., Cash, B. D., Pimentel, M., & Porter, C. K. (2013). "Pathogen-specific risk of celiac disease following bacterial causes of foodborne illness: a retrospective cohort study." *Digestive Diseases and Sciences*, *58*(11), 3242–3245.

Rodrigo, L., Blanco, I., Bobes, J., & de Serres, F. J. (2013). "Clinical impact of a gluten-free diet of health-related quality of life in seven fibromyalgia syndrome patients with associated celiac disease." *BMC Gastroenterology*, *13*(1), 157. doi: 10.1186/1471-230X-13-157.

Rostami, K., Steegers, E. A., Wong, W. Y., Braat, D. D., & Steegers-Theunissen, R. P. (2001). "Coeliac disease and reproductive disorders: a neglected association." *European Journal of Obstetrics and Gynecology and Reproductive Biology*, *96*(2), 146–149.

Rubio-Tapia, A., Hill, I. D., Kelly, C. P., Calderwood, A. H., & Murray, J. A. (2013). ACG clinical guidelines: diagnosis and management of celiac disease. *The American Journal of Gastroenerology*, *108*(5), 656–676; quiz 677.doi: 10.1038/ajg.2013.79.

Sanchez-Albisua, I., Wolf. J., Neu, A., Geiger, H., Wascher, I., & Stern M. (2005). "Coeliac disease in children with type I diabetes mellitus: the effect of the gluten-free diet." *Diabetes Medicine*, *22* (8), 1079–1082.

Siegel, B. (1998). *Prescriptions for Living*. New York, NY: HarperCollins.

Soni, S., & Badawy, S. Z. (2010). "Celiac disease and its effect on human reproduction: a review." *The Journal of Reproductive Medicine*, *55*(1–2), 3–8. Review.

Volta, U., Caio, G., Tovoli, F., & DeGiorgio R. (2013). "Non-celiac gluten sensitivity: questions still to be answered despite increasing awareness." *Cellular Molecular Immunology, 10*(5), 383–392. doi: 10.1038/cmi.2013.28

Woodward, J. (2013). "The management of refractory coeliac disease." *Therapeutic Advances in Chronic Disease, 4*(2), 77–90. doi: 10.1177/2040622312473174.

Zebrowska, A., Narbutt, J., Sysa-Jedrzejowska, A., Kobos, J., & Waszczkowska, E. 2005. "The imbalance between mettallo-proteinases and their tissue inhibitors is involved in the pathogenesis of dermatitis herpetiformis." *Mediators of Inflammation, 2005*(6), 373–379.

Zugna D., Richiardi, L., Akre, O., Stephansson, O., & Ludvisson, J. F. (2010). "A nationwide population-based study to determine whether coeliac disease is associated with infertility." *Gut, 59*(11), 1471–1475. doi: 10.1136/gut.2010.219030.

Glossary

Anemia Reduction below normal in the number of red cells or quantity of hemoglobin that occurs when (a) blood production is disturbed, (b) there is blood loss, (c) there is poor or a lack of iron absorption.

Antibodies Cells that the body develops when it feels it is being attacked. An antibody is a protein used by the immune system to identify and neutralize foreign objects such as bacteria and viruses. Each antibody recognizes a specific antigen unique to its target. Production of antibodies is referred to as the humoral immune system.

Aphthous stomatitis Sores in the oral mucosa commonly called canker sores. (Not caused by the herpes simplex virus.)

Arrhythmia Abnormal heart rate.

Celiac/coeliac disease Also referred to as celiac sprue, gluten-sensitive enteropathy, and nontropical sprue. Symptoms include one or more of the following: gas, abdominal pain, bloating, chronic diarrhea, pale foul-smelling stools, weight loss/weight gain, fatigue, anemia, bone or joint pain, osteoporosis/osteopenia, behavioral changes, tingling numbness in legs, muscle cramps, seizures, missed menstrual periods, infertility, recurrent miscarriage, delayed growth (children), failure to thrive (infants), aphthous ulcers (sores in the mouth).

Constipation   Infrequent or difficult evacuation of feces (stool).

Crohn's disease   An inflammation of the digestive tract. Most commonly affects the lower part of the small intestine called the ilium. The swelling extends deep into the lining of the affected area (all layers may be involved). Also called ileitis or enteritis. Symptoms include: abdominal pain, diarrhea, bloating, weight loss and/or bleeding.

Dental enamel hypoplasia   Loss of enamel on teeth due to malabsorption of calcium.

Dermatitis herpetiformis   Skin condition that occurs in 25% of CD patients. The skin eruptions are extremely itchy and are a manifestation of the damage that is happening in the small intestine.

Diabetes mellitus type 1   Usually called juvenile diabetes which is a condition requiring insulin to regulate the blood sugar.

Diabetes mellitus type 2   Common onset is over 40 years of age. Controlled with hypoglycemic medication and diet.

Diarrhea   Abnormal and frequent liquid evacuation of feces (stool).

Down syndrome   A chromosomal condition associated with mental retardation, characteristic facial expressions, and poor muscle tone. Increased risk of other physical conditions.

Endomysial antibodies   Antibodies produced when the gluten in grains are introduced into an individual with CD.

Endoscopy   Procedure that allows the gastroenterologist to examine and biopsy the esophagus, stomach, duodenum, and small intestine by using a tube (scope) with a light on it.

Enriched   Adding back nutrients lost during the processing of the food product.

Fortified   Adding nutrients that are not present in the original product.

Gliadin   A protein complex found in wheat that produces antibodies in an individual with CD.

Gluten ataxia   A loss of balance condition of CD which is caused by the antibodies tissue transglutaminase six (tTG6).

Gluten contamination elimination diet (GCED)   A detailed list of ingested foods that can identify what foods create symptoms and determine gluten contamination in the diet.

Gluten-free diet (GFD)   A diet that contains no known proteins of wheat, barley, and/or rye.

Gluten-sensitive enteropathy   A diagnosis frequently used for CD.

Glutenin   A protein found in wheat.

Hemoglobin   An iron-containing red blood cell that functions to transport oxygen from the lungs to the tissues of the body.

Hordein   A protein complex found in barley that produces antibodies in an individual with CD.

Hypochondria (hypochondriac)   Severe anxiety about one's health associated with numerous and varying symptoms that cannot be attributed to disease.

Immunochromatographic assay   A highly accurate new laboratory test that is showing promise in diagnosing CD.

Iron deficiency anemia   Caused by iron deficiency either by blood loss, malabsorption of iron in the small intestine, or disturbance of blood production.

Irritable bowel syndrome   An inflammation of the intestine that can occur in any part of the intestinal tract from various causes. Symptoms include: diarrhea, abdominal bloating, abdominal pain, and constipation.

Lactose intolerance   Inability to digest lactose, which is the sugar found in milk. Results in abdominal pain, bloating, gas, and possible diarrhea.

Lupus erythematosus (SLE)   Autoimmune disease that is a generalized connective tissue disorder, usually involving several body systems.

Malabsorption   Any condition that prevents nutrients from being absorbed from foods into the digestive tract.

Multiple sclerosis   An autoimmune disease in which there are lesions in the central nervous system causing numbness, speech problems, and visual problems. It has periods of remission and is a long-term condition.

Multisystem disorder   More than one system in the body is affected. In CD, the gastrointestinal tract is involved; however, the skin, brain, and other areas of the body may be involved.

Non-responsive celiac disease (NRCD) When symptoms persist while on the GFD.

Osteoporosis Calcium deficiency that results in bones becoming porous and increasing a risk of fracture.

Peripheral neuropathy Loss of feeling in the fingers or toes as a result of nerve endings dying.

Prolamines A protein complex found in grains that produces antibodies in an individual with CD.

Refractory celiac disease (RCD) Persistent symptoms and signs of malabsorption after gluten exclusion for 12 months with ongoing villous atrophy.

Seculin A protein complex found in rye that produces antibodies in an individual with CD.

Sjögren's syndrome Autoimmune disease that occurs in middle-aged or older women. Symptoms include: dryness of the mouth, inflammation of the eyes, and enlargement of the parotid glands.

Small intestine The area of the digestive tract between the stomach and large intestine. It contains the villi (or folds) that absorb most nutrients.

Sprue A term formerly used for celiac disease (celiac sprue).

Tissue transglutaminase A family of enzymes that are specific and sensitive to the antibodies produced by CD. (tTG 2 in the gut, tTG 3 in the skin, and tTG 6 in the nervous system.)

Turner syndrome Chromosomal condition that affects development in females.

Ulcerative colitis Inflammation and sores in lining of the rectum and colon. Symptoms include: diarrhea, abdominal pain, anemia, fatigue, loss of appetite, weight loss, rectal bleeding, skin lesions, joint pain, and growth failure (children).

Villi The small hair-like projections in the small intestine that absorb nutrients from food.

Williams syndrome Developmental disorder that affects many parts of the body. Mild to moderate mental retardation, unique personal characteristics, distinctive facial features, and heart and blood vessel problems.

Wireless capsule endoscopy A miniaturized camera that is swallowed and remotely visualizes the intestinal tract.

Xanthan gum Substance added to gluten-free baked products to add elasticity to the dough.

Index

About the Authors

Sylvia Llewelyn Bower, RN, lives with celiac disease, has been a practicing nurse for 50 years, and has been certified in Nursing Administration and as a Case Manager. She has participated in the Gluten-Free Gang, one of the first celiac disease support groups, for over 16 years. She has been a member of the Ohio Nurses Association and has spoken multiple times at the National Annual Celiac Conference. She is the author of *What Nurses Know...Gluten-Free Lifestyle* and has published articles in a variety of media outlets including the Gluten Intolerance Group Magazine.

Mary Kay Sharrett, SM, RD, LD, CNSD, is a clinical dietitian at Columbus Children's Hospital in Columbus, Ohio. She is the clinical liaison to the Columbus Children's Hospital Gluten-Free Gang Support Group.

Steve Plogsted, PharmD, is a pharmacist at Columbus Children's Hospital in Columbus, Ohio. He specializes in the prescription and over-the-counter medication needs of patients with celiac disease. He has spoken at numerous regional and national conferences on the topic of medication and the celiac patient.